Lasers in Medicine
AN INTRODUCTORY GUIDE

Lasers in Medicine
AN INTRODUCTORY GUIDE

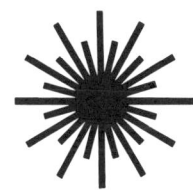

Second edition

Gregory T. Absten
BSc, MA

President of Advanced Laser Services Corporation, Columbus, Ohio — an independent laser consulting and technical services firm. Formerly Instructor in Laser Surgery at the University of Cincinnati Medical College and Scientific Fellow of the American Society for Laser Medicine and Surgery.

and

Stephen N. Joffe
BSc, MB, ChB, MD, FRCS, FCS, FACS

Professor of Surgery at the University of Cincinnati Medical Center and President of Laser Centers of America, Inc.

London
CHAPMAN AND HALL

First published in 1985 by
Chapman and Hall Ltd
11 New Fetter Lane, London EC4P 4EE

Distributed exclusively in the USA by
Lasers Centers of America
Suite 1140, 250 East 5th St
Cincinnati, Ohio 45202, USA

Second edition 1989

© 1985, 1989 G.T. Absten and S.N. Joffe

Set in 10/12pt Parlament by
Leaper & Gard Ltd, Bristol
Printed in Great Britain by
The University Press, Cambridge

ISBN 0 412 30870 3

This paperback edition is sold subject to the condition that it shall not, by way of trade or otherwise, be lent, resold, hired out, or otherwise circulated without the publisher's prior consent in any form of binding or cover other than that in which it is published and without a similar condition including this condition being imposed on the subsequent purchaser.

All rights reserved. No part of this book may be reprinted or reproduced, or utilized in any form or by any electronic, mechanical or other means, now known or hereafter invented, including photocopying and recording, or in any information storage and retrieval system, without permission in writing from the publisher.

British Library Cataloguing in Publication Data

Absten, Gregory, T.
  Lasers in medicine. — 2nd ed.
  1. medicine. Use of lasers
  I. Title   II. Joffe, Stephen N.
  610'.28
  ISBN 0 412 30870 3

Library of Congress Cataloging-in-Publication Data

Absten, Gregory T.
  Lasers in medicine: an introductory guide/
     Gregory T. Absten,
  Stephen N. Joffe. – [2nd ed.]
       p.   cm.
  Bibliography: p.
  Includes index.
  ISBN 0 412 30870 3
  1. Lasers in medicine.   I. Joffe, Stephen N.   II. Title.
R857.L37A27 1988
610'.28–dc19   88-10843
                                                  CIP

Contents

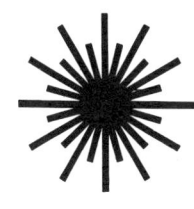

	Acknowledgements	vii
	Preface	ix
	Glossary	xi
1	**Simplified Physics**	1
	Properties of waves	1
	Where does light come from?	3
	Special properties of laser light	7
	The laser medium	9
	What are sealed tube lasers (Carbon dioxide)?	10
	Energy concepts	12
	Optical concepts	12
2	**Laser–Tissue Interactions**	16
3	**Properties of Individual Lasers**	22
	The carbon dioxide (CO_2) laser	22
	The argon laser	23
	KTP (Potassium Titanyl Phosphate) laser	24
	The Nd:YAG (Neodymium:Yttrium Aluminum Garnet) laser	25
	The dye laser	25
	The excimer laser	26
4	**Laser Beam Delivery Systems**	27
	Carbon dioxide lasers	27
	Argon and KTP lasers	29
	Dye lasers	30
	Excimer lasers	30
	Nd:YAG lasers	30
	Aiming beams	33
5	**Overview of Clinical Applications**	34
	Gynecology	35
	Otorhinolaryngology	37
	Pulmonary medicine	38

	Neurosurgery	39
	Dermatology and plastic surgery	41
	Gastroenterology	42
	Urology	43
	Oral surgery and dentistry	45
	General surgery	45
	Orthopedics	46
	Ophthalmology	46
	Vascular surgery	49
	Photodynamic therapy	50
	Laserthermia® or interstitial local hyperthermia	53
6	**Laser Safety**	54
	General points	54
	Carbon dioxide lasers	57
	Nd:YAG lasers	59
	Argon and KTP lasers	61
	Further Reading	63
	Index	65

Color plates appear between pages 46 and 47

Acknowledgements

I would like to thank all the physicians, nurses, and others I have worked with over the years, in hospitals throughout the United States and Europe, for their professional support and encouragement. No matter how much I teach, I always feel as if I am learning new things from those I am instructing.

Thanks to Doctor James McCaughan Jr for the use of Photodynamic Therapy illustrations and for help with that section of the book.

I especially want to acknowledge my children, Eric and Nicole, for letting their dad be a 'laser-head' most of the time.

Parts of this book appear in an article entitled *Fundamentals of Laser Surgery*, by G.T. Absten, published by Advanced Laser Services Corporation, Columbus, Ohio, USA.

G.T. Absten

Preface

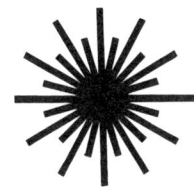

In every area of human endeavor, technology has opened the door for new advancements to occur. Much of the progress in medicine over the last few years is due, in large part, to new technological tools made available to clinicians and researchers. Laser is an expanding technological discipline in medicine that will ultimately contribute to a broad and rapid expansion of both diagnostic and treatment procedures.

Laser is to light what music is to noise. Those physicians who wish to be most successful in the application of this technology, to the benefit of their patient, will learn of the subtle interactions of light with tissue.

No technology is good or bad in itself. It is only in the choices we make, in when and how to apply that technology, that it gains its moral value. The use of lasers in medicine has some very definite advantages in the surgical and medical treatment of a variety of disorders.

At the same time we must all be careful to not perpetuate the myth of lasers in medicine. Vastly overstated claims of the value of 'laser surgery' have been held out to the general public, resulting in health care being sought on the basis of laser availability.

It is important to remember that, in the practice of medicine, it is the physicians who are the prime determinants of the quality of health care, and not the tools they choose to use. The laser can be a wonderful tool when used by an experienced, well trained physician.

This book has been written to provide a basic introduction to the use of lasers in medicine – what they are, how they work, and what they can do for the patient. It assumes only a basic scientific background in the reader, and has many simple and clear diagrams. It should be excellent as an overview of the activity in lasers in medicine to physicians, medical students, nurses, biomedical engineers, patients and the interested public. The science of light is a fascinating topic which is easily understood from a conceptual point of view.

An encyclopedic glossary of laser terms is included which, in itself, provides a quick, easy introduction to medical laser concepts.

The physical principle on which lasers are based developed from Einstein's theories in the early 1900s, though the first laser device was not produced until the 1960s. Einstein had a quest – to show that the four basic forces of the universe are simply different faces of the same singular force. The single force of the universe – that is the ultimate quest of all of physics, and of philosophy.

Glossary

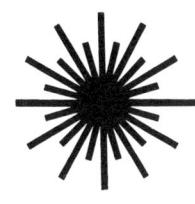

Ablation	volume removal of tissue by vaporization.
Absorption	uptake of light energy by tissue, converting it into heat.
Absorption coefficient	factor describing light's ability to be absorbed. Optical properties of different tissues alter the absorption.
Active medium	(laser medium) the material used to emit the laser light.
Aiming beam	a HeNe laser (or other light source) used as a guide light. Used coaxially with infrared or other invisible light.
Amplitude	the maximum height of a wave. Implies power.
Argon	the gas used as a laser medium. It emits blue/green light at 488 and 515 nm.
Articulated arm	a CO_2 laser delivery device consisting of hollow metal tubes with joints which allow the 'arm' to move. Mirrors are located at each joint to reflect the laser beam.
Attenuation	decreasing the intensity (power) of light as it passes through a medium.
Biostimulation	the use of low power light (milliwatts), usually laser, to stimulate metabolic activity on a subcellular level. Experimentally examined for pain relief and wound healing.
Carbon dioxide	(CO_2) molecule used as a laser medium. Emits far infrared light at 10600 nm (10.6μ). Lasers are made as sealed tube, or flowing gas units.
Cautery	achieving hemostasis of bleeding vessels,

usually by heat from laser or electrosurgical units. Contrasts with laser induced protein coagulation.

Chromophore — optically active (colored) material in tissue which acts as the target for laser light.

Coagulation — destruction of tissue by heat without physically removing it.

Coherence — orderliness of wave patterns by being in phase in time and space.

Combiner mirror — the mirror in a laser which combines two or more wavelengths into a coaxial beam, i.e. CO_2 and HeNe beams.

Contact probe — synthetic ceramic material, like sapphire, used with laser fibers to allow touch of tissue with the probe, intensifying its effects, and allowing cutting, vaporizing, or coagulation of tissue at relatively low powers and high degree of control.

Continuous wave — (CW) constant, steady state delivery of laser power.

Collimation — ability of the laser beam to not spread (low divergence) with distance.

Dichroic filter — filter that allows selective transmission of colors.

DHE — dihematoporphyrin ether. A photosensitizing agent used in PDT. DHE is a more refined form of HpD.

Diffuser — an optical device or material that homogenizes the output of light causing a very smooth, even distribution over the area affected.

Dosimetry — measuring the amount (joules) and intensity (watts/cm^2) of light delivered to tissue.

Electron — negatively charged particle of an atom.

Electromagnetic spectrum — the span of frequencies (wavelengths) considered to be light – from radio and TV waves to gamma and cosmic rays.

Endoscope — an instrument inserted into the body through an orifice (either existing or surgical) that allows viewing and manipulation of tissue.

Glossary xiii

	May be rigid or flexible.
Energy	expressed in joules (watt-seconds)
Excimer	'excited dimer'. A gas mixture used as the basis of lasers emitting ultraviolet light.
Excitation	energizing a material into a state of population inversion.
Femtoseconds	10^{-15} seconds. Shorter than picosecond or nanosecond.
Fiberoptics	a system of flexible quartz or glass fibers with internal reflective surfaces that pass light through thousands of glancing reflections. Many hundreds or thousands of individual fibers are needed to transmit an image, but only single fibers are used to transmit laser light during treatment.
Focal point	that distance from the focusing lens where the laser beam has the smallest spot diameter and hence greatest intensity.
Gated pulse	a discontinuous burst of laser light, made by timing (gating) a continuous wave output – usually in fractions of a second.
Gaussian curve	normal statistical curve showing a peak with even distribution on either side. May either be a sharp peak with steep sides, or a blunt peak with shallower sides. Used to show power distribution in a beam. The concept is important in controlling the geometry of the laser impact.
Hemostasis	the ability to stop bleeding.
HeNe	helium neon. A laser producing low power (milliwatts) red light (630 nm) used as a guide light for infrared lasers, or experimentally for biostimulation.
Hologram	a three dimensional picture made by interference patterns created by the coherence of laser light. Created as transmission, reflection or integral holograms.
HpD	hematoporphyrin derivative. A photosensitizing drug used with photodynamic therapy as a treatment for cancer.

Impact size	the size crater or width of incision left by a laser impact. Related to spot size of the beam, except impact size varies depending on how the energy is applied.
Ionizing radiation	radiation commonly associated with X-Ray, that is of a high enough energy to cause DNA damage with no direct, immediate thermal effect. Contrasts with non-ionizing radiation of surgical lasers.
Irradiance	*see* Power density.
Joule	a unit of energy. Laser powers are sometimes described in joules per second. A power of 1 joule per second is known as 1 watt and is the rate of energy delivery.
KTP	potassium titanyl phosphate. A crystal used to change the wavelength of a Nd:YAG ;laser from 1060 nm (infrared) to 532 nm (green).
Laser	Light Amplification by the Stimulated Emission of Radiation. A device that produces intense beams of pure colors of light.
Laser medium	(active medium) material used to emit the laser light and for which the laser is named.
Laser surgeon	no such thing; but some surgeons do use lasers to advantage as surgical instruments.
Metastable state	the state of an atom, just below a higher excited state, which an electron occupies momentarily before destabilizing and emitting light.
Micromanipulator (microslad)	device attached to a microscope that controls delivery of the laser beam into the microscopic field of view. In non-ophthalmic surgery, they are most commonly used with CO_2 lasers, then with argon and KTP, and least with Nd:YAG lasers.
Microprocessor	a digital chip (computer) that operates and monitors some lasers.
Mode	a term used to describe how the power of a laser beam is distributed within the geometry of the beam. Also used to describe the

Glossary xv

	operating mode of a laser such as continuous or pulsed.
Mode-locking	a process similar to Q-switching except that the pulses produced are even shorter (about 10^{-12} second) and emerge in short trains of pulses instead of singularly. It is usually achieved with a dye cell.
Monochromaticity	waves are monochromatic when they are all of the same wavelength (color).
Nanometer	abbreviated nm – a measure of length. One nm equals 10^{-9} meter, and is the usual measure of light wavelength. Visible light ranges from about 400 nm in the purple to about 750 nm in the deep red.
Nanosecond	10^{-9} (one billionth) of a second. Longer than a picosecond or femtosecond, but shorter than a microsecond. Associated with Q-switched ophthalmic Nd:YAG lasers.
Neodymium	the rare earth element that is the active element in a Nd:YAG laser.
Nd:YAG	neodymium:yttrium aluminum garnet. A mineral crystal used as a laser medium to produce 1060 nm light.
Nonlinear effect	not a normal, linear temperature rise induced by laser. Refers to the plasma 'spark' and snap created by the Q-switched Nd:YAG laser.
Optical breakdown	plasma formation by stripping electrons off atoms/molecules. Caused by high laser energy densities and used to create a 'spark'. Used in ophthalmology with Q-switched or mode-locked Nd.YAG lasers to cut membranes.
Optical cavity (resonator)	space in between the laser mirrors where lasing action occurs.
Output coupler	the partially transmissive mirror that allows laser output from the optical cavity.
PDT	photodynamic therapy. The use of photo-sensitizing drugs, activated by certain pure colors of light produced by the laser, to

achieve selective tissue destruction. Its current major use is investigationally as a selective treatment for cancer.

Phase — waves are in phase with each other when all the troughs and peaks coincide and are 'locked' together. The result is a reinforced wave of increased amplitude (brightness).

Photocoagulation — tissue coagulation caused by light (laser).

Photodisruption — creating an acoustical shock wave, through Q-switching or mode-locking, to gently 'snap' apart membranes. This is a 'cold cutting' technique with laser. Ophthalmologists use the Q-switched Nd:YAG to photodisrupt an opacified posterior capsule secondary to cataract surgery.

Photon — the basic particle of light.

Picosecond — 10^{-12} seconds. Longer than a femtosecond but shorter than a nanosecond. Associated with mode-locked ophthalmic Nd:YAG lasers.

Plasma — the fourth state of matter in which electrons have been stripped off the atoms. The extremely high internal temperature expands rapidly setting up an acoustical shock wave. Usually experienced as a lightning bolt (plasma) and resulting thunderclap (shock wave).

Plasma shield — the ability of plasma to stop transmission of laser light.

Pockel's cell — an electro-optical crystal used to achieve a Q-switch.

Population inversion — a state in which a substance has been energized, or excited, so that more atoms or molecules are in a higher given excited state than in a lower resting state. This is a necessary prerequisite for lasing action.

Power — the rate of energy delivery expressed in watts (joules per second).

Power density — (irradiance) the amount of energy concentrated into a spot of particular size. It is

	expressed in watts per square centimeter and is the brightness of the spot.
Pulse	a discontinuous burst of laser as opposed to a continuous beam. A true pulse achieves higher peak powers than that attainable in a continuous wave output – usually pulsed in microseconds or shorter. (*See also* Gated pulse).
Spot size	the mathematical measurement of a focused laser spot. In a TEM_{00} beam it is the area that contains 86% of the incident power. This is the 'optical' spot size and does not necessarily indicate the size of the laser crater that will be made. The latter is the impact size.
Superpulse	an operating moe on the CO_2 laser describing a fast pulsing output (250–1000 times per second), with peak powers per pulse higher than the maximum attainable in the continuous wave mode. Average powers of superpulse (speed of tissue removal) are always lower than the maximum in continuous wave.
Thermal relaxation time	the rate at which a structure can conduct heat. When pulse times of a laser are shorter than the time required for heat to spread out of a target, the heat damage will be confined to that target.
Tunable dye laser	a laser using a jet of liquid dye, pumped by another laser or flashlamps, to produce various colors of light. The color of light may be tuned by adjusting optical tuning elements and/or changing the dye used. Common medical applications are with the 630 nm continuous wave red, and the pulsed 577 nm yellow and 504 nm green.
Q-switching	switching the 'quality' of a resonator, producing very high peak powers (millions of watts) but for very short bursts (nanoseconds) – usually achieved with a pockel's cell. This creates a 'sparking' and shock wave

	effect (*see* Photodisruption; Plasma and Mode-locking).
X-ray	a very short wavelength of light, producing ionization effects commonly associated with radiation hazards. Not a problem with surgical laser units.

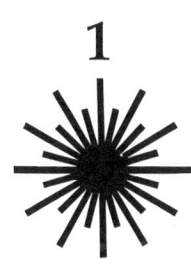

1 Simplified Physics

The word LASER is an acronym for Light Amplification by the Stimulated Emission of Radiation. Visible light is only one small portion of the electromagnetic spectrum (Fig. 1). Although the exact nature of light is still not understood, it does show properties both of discrete particles (photons) and waves. For the purposes of understanding the electromagnetic spectrum and lasers, we will primarily look at light in terms of its wave characteristics. A wave is characterized by four quantities: wavelength, amplitude, frequency and velocity (Fig. 2).

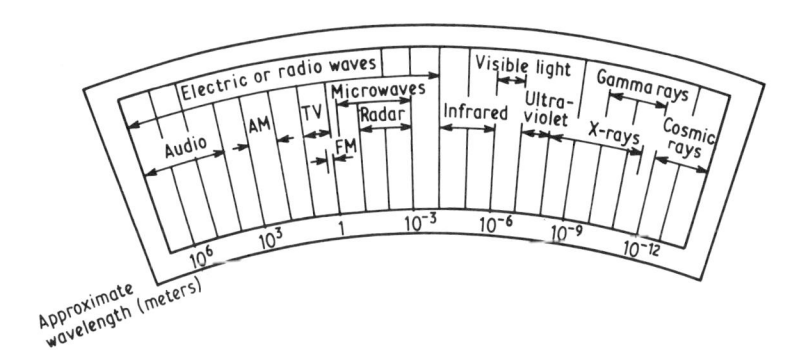

Fig.1 The electromagnetic spectrum, showing the wide range of wavelengths from the very short cosmic rays to the very long radio waves.

Properties of waves

Wavelength

The wavelength is the distance between two successive crests, or any other two points on the same parts of the wave. The color of

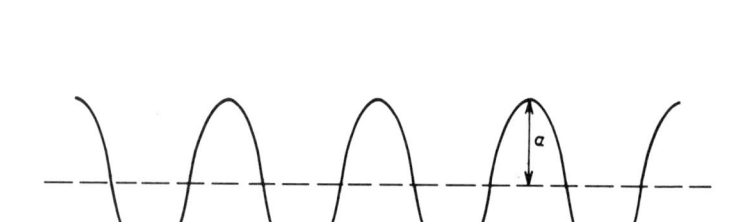

Fig. 2 The basic properties of a wave. The diagram shows a wave of velocity v, wavelength λ and amplitude a.

visible light is determined by its wavelength, which is measured in fractions of a meter known as nanometers (nm). One nm is equal to 10^{-9} m. Our eyes are designed to see only a small portion of the spectrum. Visible light waves have wavelengths in the range of about 385–760 nm (Fig. 1). More energy is associated with shorter wavelengths (blues) than with longer wavelengths (reds).

Amplitude

The amplitude is the height of the wave with maximum displacement from the zero position. Like an ocean wave, the greater the amplitude the more the power. In the case of light, the greater the amplitude the brighter the beam.

Velocity

The velocity of electromagnetic waves is a constant in a given medium, and is equal to about 186,000 miles/second or about 300,000 km/second, in a vacuum. The unique characteristic of light is that the speed of light is always constant in all frames of reference. In this sense its speed is an absolute and is further explained in Einstein's theory of relativity.

Frequency

The frequency is the number of waves passing a given point per second, and is expressed in cycles/second, or Hertz (Hz). The shorter the wavelength, the higher the frequency, since more waves will be able to pass a given point in a certain time.

Some further properties of waves also need to be considered.

Phase

Waves (of the same wavelength) are in phase when all the troughs and all the peaks are opposite each other. If two such waves meet, the result is a reinforced wave of double the amplitude (increased brightness). Conversely, if the waves are out of phase (troughs opposite peaks), then the result is a disappearance of the wave (Fig. 3).

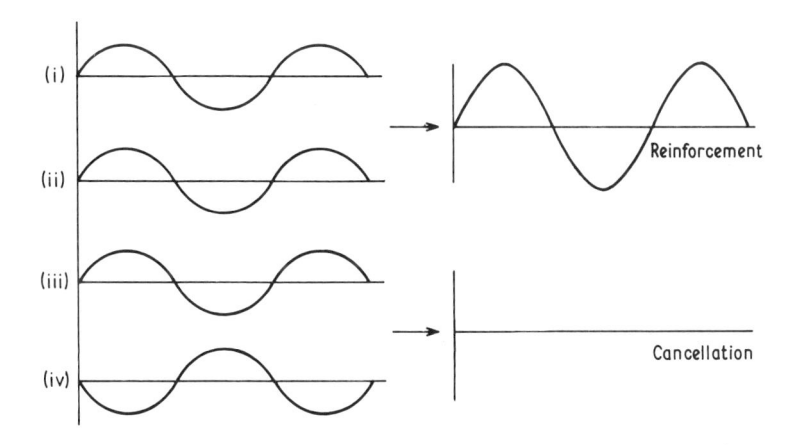

Fig. 3 Phase. Waves (i) and (ii) are 'in phase' since all the troughs and all the peaks are opposite each other. The result is a reinforced wave of double the amplitude. Waves (iii) and (iv) are 'out of phase' since troughs are opposite peaks. The result is a complete cancellation.

Coherence and incoherence

Coherent light consists of unbroken waves that are of constant wavelength and have no phase differences either in time or space (temporal and spatial coherence). An analogy may be drawn between a pure musical note (coherent) and noise (incoherent).

Where does light come from?

Having considered some of the fundamental properties of light waves, we are now in a position to understand how a laser works, where its light comes from, and how this light differs fundamentally from ordinary light.

In an atom, electrons are found to occupy certain discrete energy levels or orbits. These electrons are not free to have energies between levels or to take up positions between orbits, so that when the energy level of an atom is changed, the electrons must move up or down to the next orbital level. When an atom or molecule absorbs energy, electrons move into higher orbits, but fall back to their own less energetic resting orbits almost immediately. When an electron falls to a lower energy level, there escapes a tiny burst of surplus energy — a **photon**, the basic unit of light. The energy of the photon is simply the difference in energy between the two levels involved. Energy determines the wavelength, which is the color of the light. When many atoms in a medium undergo spontaneous orbital decay, the process is known as **spontaneous emission** (Fig. 4). The decay of different atoms occurs at random. Many energy levels are involved and the light is emitted out of phase and in all directions. Different energy levels mean multiple colors of light, and all the colors combined produce white light. This is incoherent light. The 'kernels' of light travel in all different directions out of phase with one another, just like taking the lid off a popcorn popper as all the kernels begin to explode.

A substance has the potential to become a lasing medium if it can have more atoms or molecules in a high energy state than in its resting energy state. This is known as a **population inversion**. Lasers are named after the medium that produces the light, i.e. carbon dioxide, argon, etc. Different media emit characteristic colors of light which, in turn, are used for various medical applications. In most lasers, a medium of gas, liquid or crystal is energized (pumped) by a suitable source (light, electric discharge, radio frequency). The input of pumping energy raises electrons to higher energy levels in more atoms, more quickly than spontaneous decay can return them to their original level. Once there is a preponderance of these excited atoms (i.e. atoms having an electron in a higher energy level), a further process becomes probable in addition to the spontaneous emission just described. A photon from an initial spontaneous decay stimulates each excited atom in its path to emit an identical photon, in phase, of the same color and traveling in the same direction. These photons actually fuse together in time and space producing a coherent output. This is known as **stimulated emission**, each photon stimulating another energized electron to produce a further photon, until a photon cascade of growing

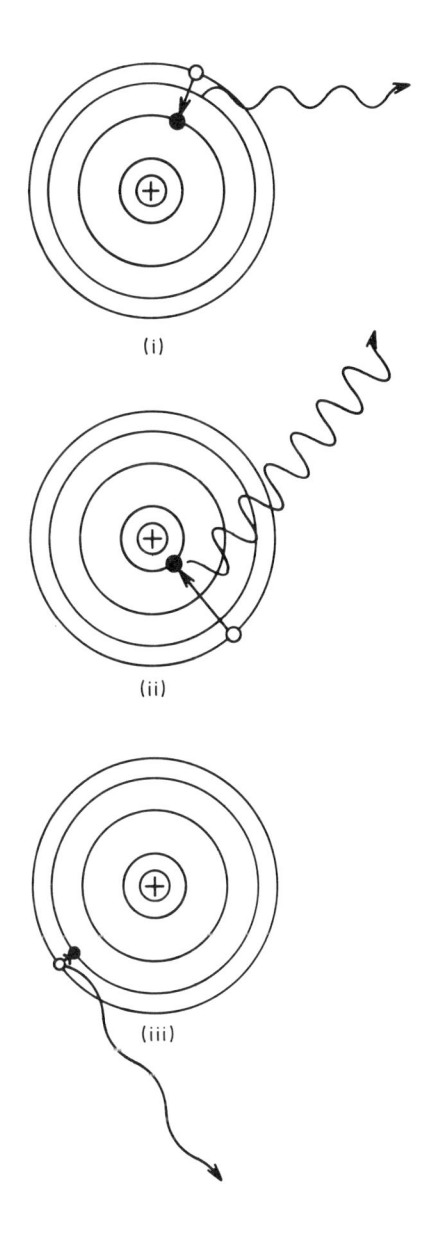

Fig. 4 Spontaneous emission. The diagrams show energized electrons in three atoms decaying back to their original orbits with the spontaneous production of a photon of light. The wavelength and amplitude of the emitted light varies according to the magnitude of the energy change, and is distributed in random directions. The overall light output is incoherent.

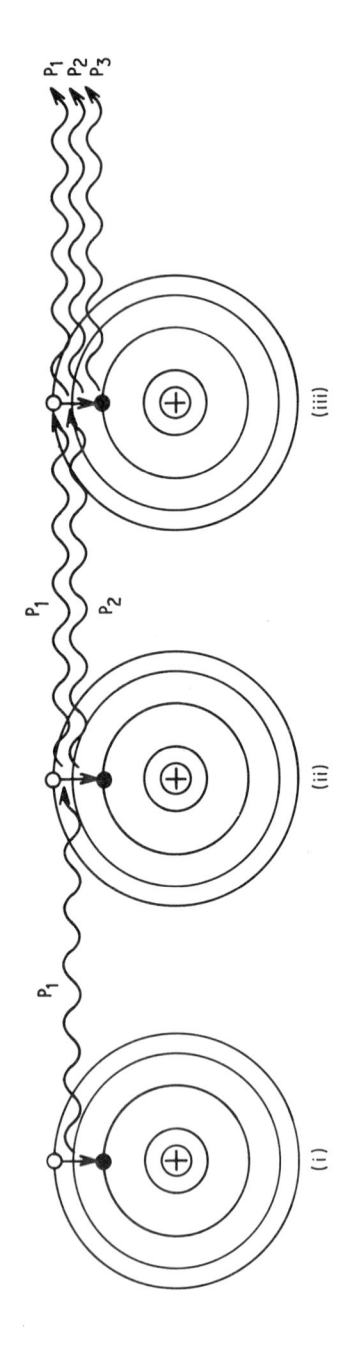

Fig. 5 Stimulated emission. The diagrams show energized electrons in three atoms in a substance which has undergone a population inversion, so that many of the atoms are in an excited state. The first atom (i) undergoes a spontaneous decay and emits a photon P_1. This interacts with a second energized atom (ii), and stimulates the emission of a second photon P_2 with precisely the same wave characteristics, and in perfect phase with P_1. Each of these identical photons can then further stimulate energized atoms to produce additional identical photons, as P_3, etc.

energy sweeps through the medium (Fig. 5). The effect is analogous to a chain of dominoes falling. The waves of light produced in this way are reflected back and forth many times by mirrors at each end of the laser chamber (Fig. 6). These mirrors perfectly face each other and form a type of 'infinity tunnel' in which the light waves are trapped and bounce back and forth at the speed of light, increasing the amplitude (power or brightness) of the wave with each pass. In medical laser systems, one of these mirrors is partially transmissive (like a two way mirror) which allows the laser beam to leak out at this end. This is the beam of laser light.

The laser beam is passed through some type of delivery system to the surgical field (Chapter 4). Fiber or articulated arms deliver the beam, and lenses or sapphire probes focus and intensify the energy. The various attachments and delivery systems determine the utility of any laser.

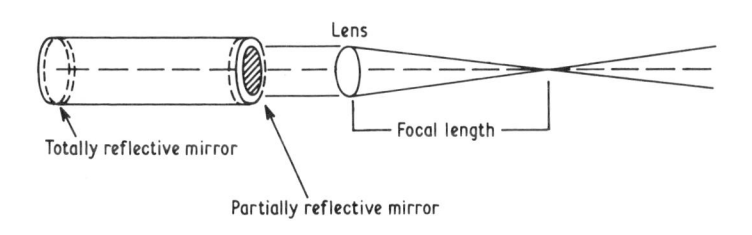

Fig. 6 Schematic diagram of laser chamber. The growing cascade of light produced by the stimulated emission is reflected back and forth between the mirrors at either end of the laser chamber until the beam leaves the chamber through the partially reflective mirror. It can then be focused by a lens, and pass into a suitable delivery system (see Chapter 4).

Special properties of laser light

Laser light differs from ordinary light in much the same way that music differs from noise. Three particular properties are responsible for this difference: coherence, collimation and monochromaticity.

Coherence

Ordinary light, from a lamp or fire, is 'incoherent', and consists of light waves radiating (shining) in all directions out of phase with one another. Since multiple wavelengths (colors) are produced, it is not even possible to phase the waves. When a handful of stones is thrown into a pool of water, the choppy wave pattern this creates on the surface is incoherent because the ripples produced by each individual stone are out of phase with one another.

Laser light is 'coherent'. Its light is also of one wavelength (color) which allows the waves to synchronize when they are phased together. When a piano tuner strikes his tuning fork, he phases the piano string to the tuning fork. The surf breaking onto the beach is also a phased wave pattern. When the peaks and troughs align, they are in phase.

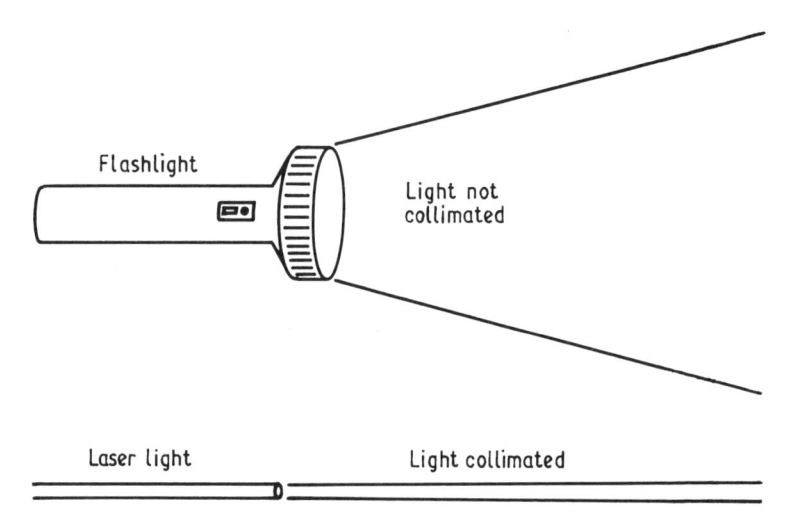

Fig. 7 Collimation. The light from a flashlight (torch) is not collimated and will spread out along the length of the beam. In contrast, the light from a laser is highly collimated, and has an insignificant spread along the length of the beam.

Collimation

A collimated beam is parallel and does not diverge, in contrast to the light from, say, a flashlight (torch) which will spread out as it travels further and further away (Fig. 7). Laser light is practically parallel, so that a laser pulse fired at the moon produces a spot half a mile wide, at a distance of 240 000 miles. For practical everyday purposes this spread is insignificant. For those of us in medicine, this means two things — that there is a minimum loss of power along the beam, and that it can be focused to intensify its effect or couple it into a slender single fiber. A laser beam can be a billion times brighter than sunlight.

Table 1 Characteristic wavelengths of light from some lasers

Laser	Color	Wavelength (nm)
Carbon dioxide	Infra-red	10600
Argon	Blue	488
	Green	515
Nd:YAG	Infra-red	1064
KTP	Green	532
Krypton	Red	647
	Yellow	568
	Green	531
Ruby	Deep red	694
Helium neon	Red	632
Gold vapor	Red	632
Copper vapor	Yellow	578
Dye laser	(variable with dyes)	
	Red	632
	Green	504
	Yellow	577
Excimers:	Ultraviolet:	
Argon fluoride		193
Krypton fluoride		248
Xenon chloride		308
Xenon chloride		351

Monochromaticity

Monochromaticity indicates that the light is all of the same wavelength (color). Ordinary light sources produce light from a hot body process. Like the glowing filament in a lamp, the light usually consists of a mixture of all possible colors in a broad range. This results in white light. All the light of the laser is concentrated in a few discrete wavelengths (frequently one) (Table 1). Lasers produce pure colors of light. Different materials emit characteristic colors.

The laser medium

A laser is usually named after its active medium, the substance which exhibits the lasing action. This can be a liquid, solid, or gas. Substances which have been used include the following:

Solids (Crystals): Ruby, Nd:YAG (Yttrium Aluminum Garnet, doped with neodymium — a rare earth element), Nd:Glass, Er:YAG

(Erbium Yag), alexandrite, Nd:GASG (Gadolinium Aluminum Scandium Garnet doped with neodymium).

Gases: Carbon dioxide, argon, krypton, helium–neon, carbon monoxide, hydrogen fluoride, argon fluoride, xenon chloride.

Liquids: Dyes of different types which allow emission of various wavelengths depending on the dye, giving rise to the name Tunable Dye laser.

Other substances have also been used, but the lasers which have found the widest applications in medicine at the moment are those based on carbon dioxide, argon, Nd:YAG, krypton and various dyes. All of these substances need to be energized into a state of population inversion. Solid and liquid lasers tend to be energized optically, usually by flash lamps or another laser, and gas lasers which tend to be energized electrically by direct current, or radio frequency (RF).

What are sealed tube lasers (Carbon dioxide)?

When the carbon dioxide gas mixture is energized and stimulated to emit its light, there is a disassociation of the molecule into carbon monoxide and a free oxygen radical, unlike argon or neodymium atoms which do not break apart (Fig. 8). The resulting molecule is no longer able to produce light. Complicating this is the fact that the electrodes in the laser tube give off contaminants which further degrades the gas mixture. In medicine, three basic configurations of carbon dioxide lasers have resulted.

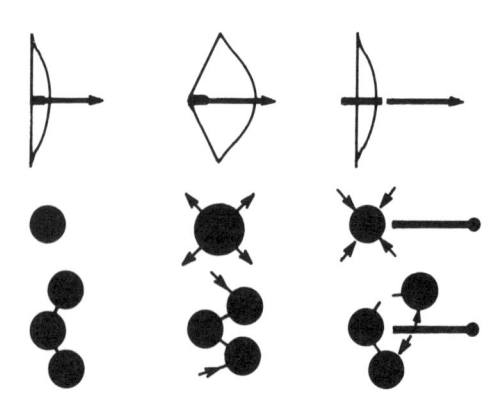

Fig. 8 Light emission from a carbon dioxide gas mixture.

Flowing gas systems

Because of the disassociation of the molecule, and electrode contamination, a flowing gas system is used to purge the tube and replenish the gas. This requires cylinders of replacement gas, pressure regulators, and a vacuum pump to draw the gas through the system. All of this adds to the maintenance, noise, and expense of operating the laser. On the other hand, flowing gas systems produce a reliable, steady output, and easily generate high powers (for medicine) of 50–100 watts. They also produce stable, low power outputs of around 1 watt.

Free space, sealed tube lasers

These are a newer generation laser tube that eliminates the need for replacement laser gas mixture, regulators and vacuum pumps. They can produce power levels comparable to flowing gas systems up to about 100 watts.

This sealed tube laser uses direct current (DC) excitation as do the flowing gas systems. The electrodes are specially treated, and catalysts and inhibitors are added to the self-contained gas mixture to retard breakdown of the gas. This allows for a sealed tube type of laser system. After several years the tubes will need to be recharged as the power begins to gradually fall from the high end.

Radio frequency (RF) waveguides

These are also sealed tube systems but instead of using direct current applied through electrodes to energize the gas they utilize a radio frequency that is transmitted transversely across the tube to excite the gas molecules, which eliminates the electrode problems. The ceramic tube of the laser is also impregnated with catalysts and inhibitors to retard breakdown of the gas. The radio frequency is contained within a waveguide structure of the laser. There is no interference with monitors or electrical equipment. RF waveguide lasers have typically produced lower power of 25 watts and under, though newer technology systems are producing outputs of up to 50 watts.

Sealed tube systems of both varieties are generally simpler to operate, quieter, and require less routine maintenance than flowing gas systems. Both flowing gas, and sealed tube systems each have their own advantages.

Energy concepts

Power is simply a measure of the **rate** of energy delivery in joules/second, and is expressed in watts. Of greater importance is the amount of power which can be focused into a spot. This **power density**, or irradiance (sometimes called spot brightness), of a laser is the number of watts/cm² of a spot, and is the single most important factor in the effective application of a laser. The surface area of the spot (spot size controlled by the surgeon in the field), and the total power in watts (set at the laser by the operator) determine the power density as follows:

$$\frac{watts \times 100}{\pi \times r^2} = watts/cm^2$$

Power density over a spot determines the rate of tissue removal within that spot. One can effectively change the size of the 'paintbrush' (spot size) without changing the overall rate of tissue removal (power density) by varying the power. The larger the spot, the greater the power required to maintain the same power density, shown as follows:

	0.6 mm spot	2.0 mm spot
1900 watts/cm²:	10 watts	60 watts

The total energy within the beam is expressed in **joules**. Power multiplied by delivery time equals the number of joules. 10 watts delivered for three seconds is 30 joules of energy. Joules describe the total energy delivered but does not by itself indicate how concentrated this dose of light is.

Fluence combines the concepts of power density (spot brightness) and dosage (joules), and is expressed in joules/cm².

Optical concepts

The focal length of the laser lens

On non-fiberoptic delivery systems (carbon dioxide lasers), lenses are interchangeable. The smaller the focal length of the lens, the smaller the spot size and the greater the power density at any given power. Carbon dioxide lasers are able to achieve spot sizes in the range 0.025–0.05 mm, but most medical systems produce spots of 0.1–0.8 mm.

The wavelength of the laser

Each laser has its own characteristic wavelength (Table 1). The shorter the wavelength, the smaller the spot which can be produced. An argon (515 nm) or KTP (Potassium Titanyl Phosphate, 532 nm) would be able to produce spots much smaller than a carbon dioxide laser (10,600 nm). However, a type of laser would be chosen for its specific effects on tissue rather than its spot size capabilities. On any type of fiberoptically delivered laser, the smallest focused spot which can be achieved is the size of the tip of the fiber, regardless of the wavelength. An argon laser delivered through a 0.4 mm fiber could not be focused any smaller than a 0.4 mm spot.

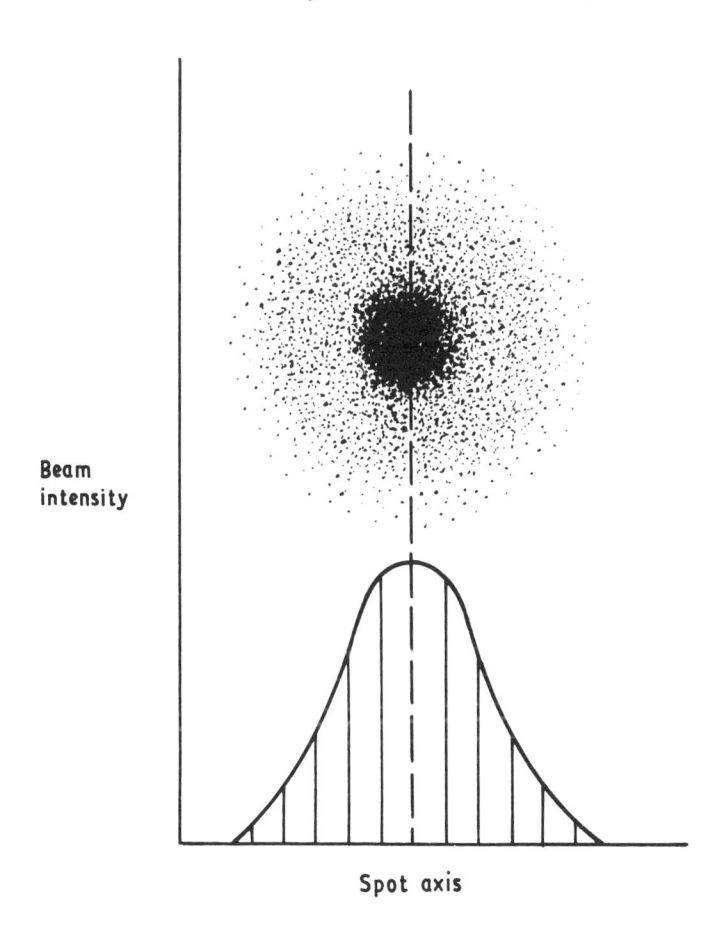

Fig.9 Mode TEM$_{00}$, with most of the power at the centre of the spot.

The mode

Mode refers to the distribution of power over the spot area, and determines the precision of the operative spot size. The technical term is Transverse Electromagnetic Mode (TEM) of the beam. The most fundamental mode, known as TEM_{00}, shows a power distribution of the spot which has most of the power at the center. A graph of beam intensity against its axis is shown in Fig. 9. This mode can be focused to the smallest spots and is the cleanest beam. Most of the medical carbon dioxide lasers produce this clean beam. This concept is not applicable to fiberoptically delivered lasers since the fiber destroys the mode structure.

When the intensity is not distributed in this fundamental mode, it is said to be in a multimode distribution. Many different mode

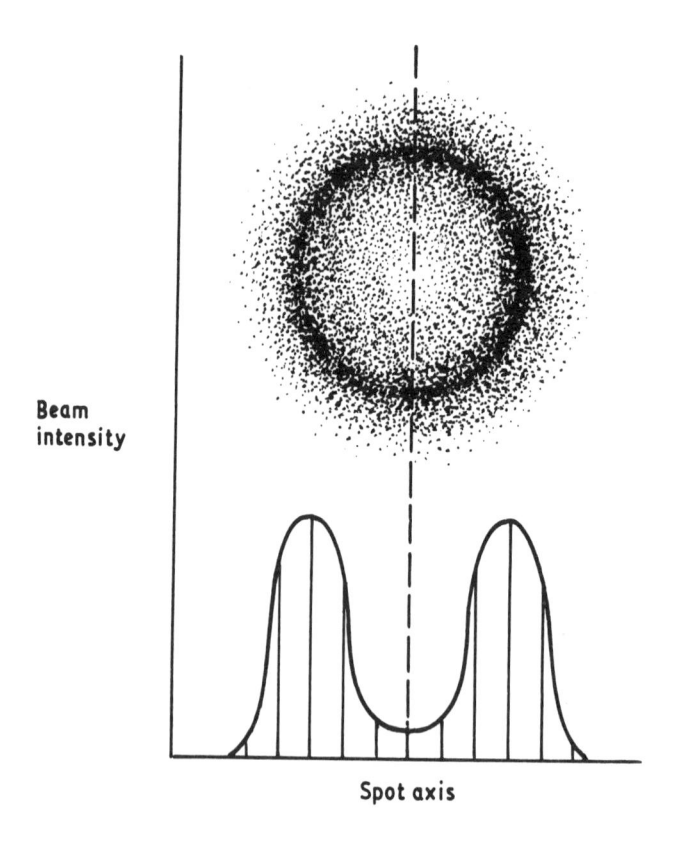

Fig. 10 Mode TEM_{01}, with a 'cold' region in the center of the spot.

structures can be present simultaneously. A common mode which occurs in the first fraction of a second of a pulse for high powered (100 watt) carbon dioxide lasers is known as TEM$_{01}$, which exhibits a cold region in the center of a doughnut shaped burn (Fig. 10).

Q-switching and mode-locking

Q-switching is a term used to describe the switching quality of a resonator, causing it to produce high peak powers but lasting for very brief intervals, frequently in nanoseconds (10^{-9} seconds). This is usually associated with ophthalmic Nd:YAG lasers, causing a spark and snap in the eye. However some other types of lasers in medicine are beginning to employ this pulsing technique, holding just short of the spark and snap. Mode-locking is also used in some ophthalmic Nd:YAG lasers, creating similar end results but through a different mechanism, resulting in a train of much shorter pulse widths, in the range of picoseconds (10^{-12} seconds).

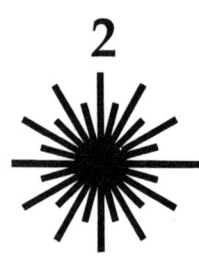

2 Laser–Tissue Interactions

The effects created by surgical lasers – namely cutting, vaporizing and coagulation – are all caused by heating of the tissue. Table 2 describes the effects on soft tissue as the temperature increases, from a laser or any other source of heat. The wavelength (color) of the laser is important only in determining how efficiently this heat transfer occurs, and over what volume of tissue. The nature of interaction of all laser light with biological tissue can be described in terms of reflection, transmission, scattering or absorption (Fig. 11).

Table 2 Absorptive heating

Temperature °C	Visual change	Biological change
100	Smoke plume	Vaporization, carbonization
90–100	Puckering	Drying
65–90	White/Grey	Protein denaturization
60–65	Blanching	Coagulation
37–60	None	Warming, welding

In order for light to heat tissue it must be absorbed. If it is reflected from or transmitted through tissue no effect will occur. If the light is scattered, it will be absorbed over a larger volume so that its effects will be more diffuse. Fig. 12 compares the relative effects of carbon dioxide, argon (or KTP), and Nd:YAG lasers. This shows the relative spread of thermal damage from the raw beam only, and ignores other important factors such as delivery systems, power densities, powers and pulse times.

As indicated, the carbon dioxide laser is the most highly

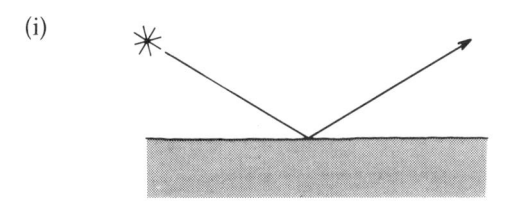

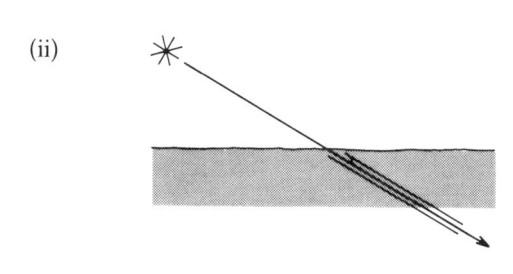

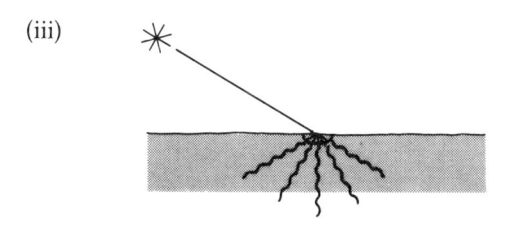

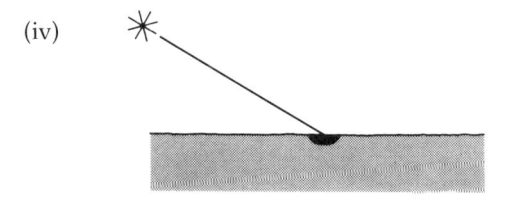

Fig. 11 (i) Reflection. A laser beam is reflected from the surface of a tissue, and has no effect.
(ii) Transmission. A laser beam is transmitted through a tissue, and has no, or only very minimal, effect.
(iii) Scattering. A laser beam is scattered by a tissue, and absorbed over a large area. Its effects are diffuse, and weakened.
(iv) Absorption. A laser beam is absorbed by a small volume of tissue, and exerts its effects within this volume.

18 Laser–Tissue Interactions

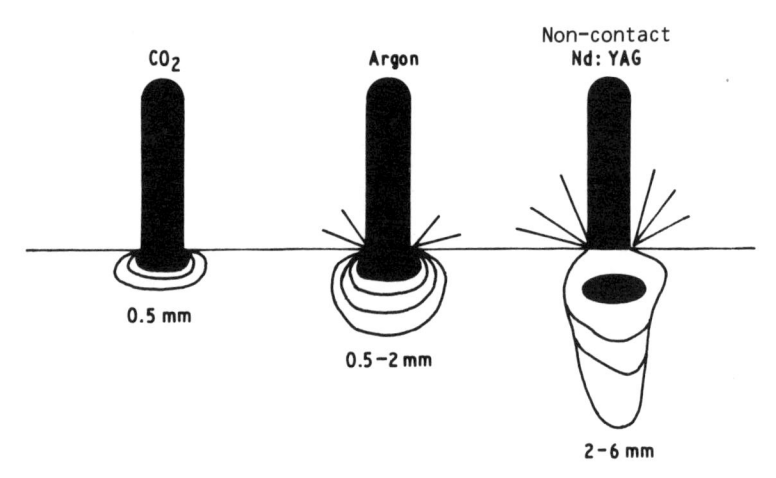

Fig. 12 Tissue reaction and depth of thermal damage of CO_2, argon and non-contact Nd:YAG lasers.

absorbed, only 30–90 microns in water, and causes the most intense heating effects – cutting and vaporization. It will coagulate tissue, but only superficially.

The Nd:YAG laser scatters its light over a broad volume of tissue causing coagulation as deep as 2–6 mm if desired. At higher power densities it will vaporize, but leaves an underlying deep coagulation beneath the base of the crater. In Chapter 4 we will look at how sapphire probes can completely change these characteristics.

The argon (488 and 515 nm) and the KTP (532 nm) lasers produce very similar if not identical tissue effects from a clinical perspective. They are generally considered superficial coagulators, causing necrosis 0.5–2.0 mm deep. At smaller spots and higher power densities they can also be used for very fine cutting, although they proceed very slowly because of their relatively low powers of around 15 watts. There are some differences in the absorption peaks of argon and KTP, and the high frequency pulsing of the KTP compared to argon. For a general understanding of tissue effects they are considered equivalent.

Vaporization of tissue occurs when cellular fluid is heated to its boiling point. The rapid rise in intracellular temperature and pressure causes an explosion of the cell, throwing off steam and cellular debris known as 'laser plume' (Fig. 13).

Soft tissue vaporizes at 100 degrees Centigrade. If the remnant carbon is allowed to build, and lasing is attempted through this carbon, the lasing point will begin to incandesce to an orange glow

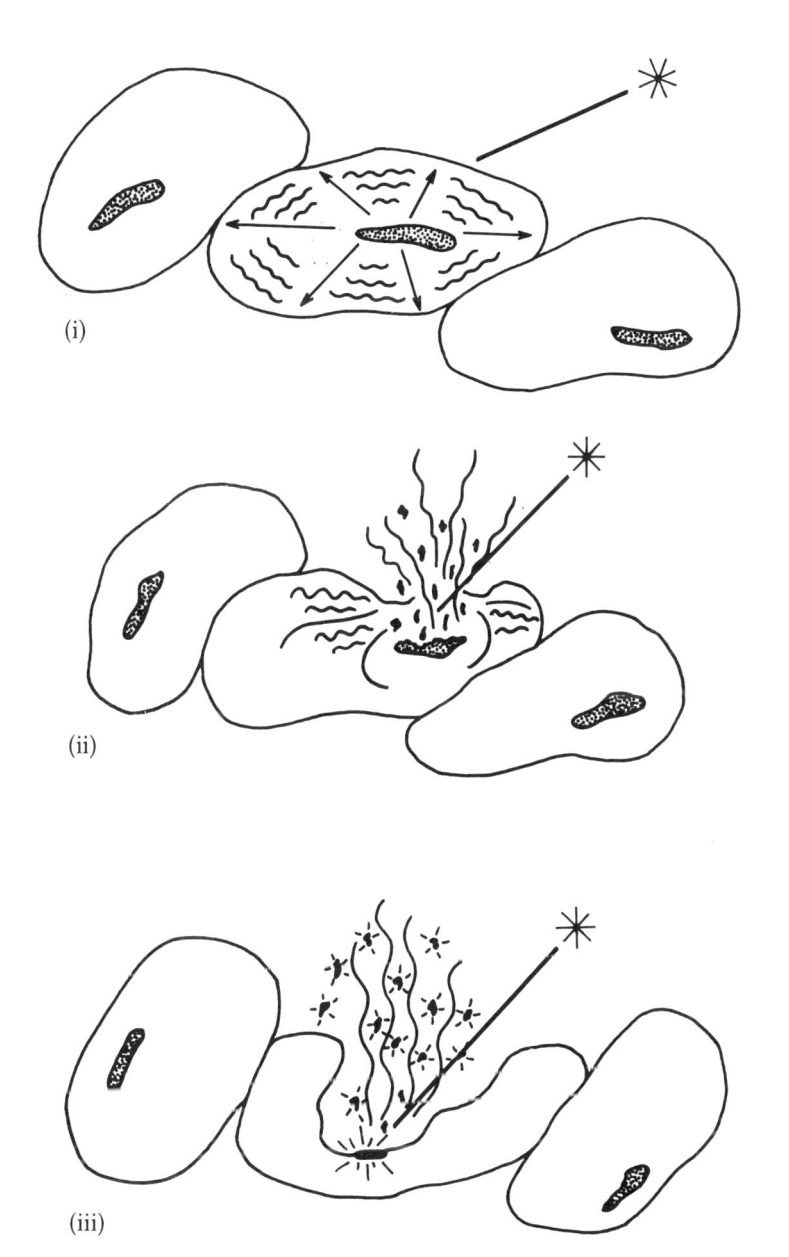

Fig. 13 (i) A cell has absorbed laser light and is heated to boiling point. The cell is destroyed.
(ii) The cell explodes, throwing off steam and cellular debris.
(iii) The steam and debris rise from the site of impact and are carbonized in the laser beam.

as tissue heats to over 1500 degrees centigrade. This would cause extensive thermal damage resulting in a branding iron type burn and concomitant scarring. It is usually created by lasing at power densities that are too low for excessive lengths of time. When concerned about potential scarring or cosmetic results, any char should be wiped away before continuing to lase over the same site.

Cutting is simply vaporizing tissue along a line, using very small spot sizes of 0.1–0.5 mm. Defocusing the beam slightly, using higher power to maintain power density, and cutting with this broader beam, results in less precision but better hemostasis for vascular areas. This is primarily done with the carbon dioxide laser.

Coagulation of tissue with laser has a broader meaning than simply achieving hemostasis. The laser has the ability to destroy cells by denaturing the protein without necessarily vaporizing it. This would be like heating egg white and seeing it turn white as it coagulates. Deep coagulation may sometimes be desirable as when treating bladder tumors. The Nd:YAG laser has the deepest coagulating abilities, followed by the argon laser. Hemostasis, or cautery, is achieved by sealing the ends of the capillaries or vessels with the laser heat, secondary to cutting or vaporizing. The greater the blood flow through a vessel, the more it acts as a heat sink, and the greater the difficulty in achieving hemostasis. Applying pressure, when possible, to slow the blood flow helps to achieve better hemostasis.

Hemostasis achieved with a laser may be similar to spray coagulation achieved with electrocautery, with the laser being more controllable and predictable, and able to work in a non-contact mode. Laser treatment may eliminate the need for electrocautery but in some cases the advantages of laser over electrosurgical coagulation have been overstated. Electrosurgery may take many different forms, from delicate coagulation with bipolar forceps, fine cutting with a micro-needle, to the charring and burning in the spray coagulation mode. Lasers cannot perform tissue excavation or snaring as electrosurgery. These modalities may complement one another.

Since bone and cartilage contain relatively little water, they vaporize differently from soft tissue. Bone has a tendency to heat as does carbon, and conducts heat into the adjacent soft tissue. To protect these tissues and limit the thermal damage, a superpulse mode is preferred with the carbon dioxide lasers. This appears as a continuous beam, but is actually cycling on and off from 250–1000 times per second with high peak powers (250–500 watts) on each spike. This allows a cooler cutting of the bone or cartilage. Most carbon dioxide lasers offer some variety of superpulse. Though this modality is useful, claims of the commercial advantages of varying different superpulse parameters are exaggerated. Bone may also need to be continuously irrigated to prevent flaming. It must be said that the cutting of bone with a laser is not entirely satisfactory. Investigators are examining the use of the 193 nm argon fluoride and 2.94 μ Er:YAG lasers for this purpose because of their non-thermal type of cutting.

3 Properties of Individual Lasers

The carbon dioxide (CO$_2$) laser

The carbon dioxide laser has been the primary instrument for surgery, with the contact Nd:YAG quickly gaining ground. Unlike the argon or KTP lasers, the specific absorption of its 10,600 nm light by water in soft tissue is independent of tissue color. The high degree of absorption with limited lateral damage makes this laser a precise surgical instrument to cut or vaporize tissue in a no-touch technique.

As we will discuss later, the Nd:YAG laser, when used with contact probes, can achieve similar effects to the carbon dioxide laser in terms of cutting or vaporizing. Though more difficult in its operation to learn, the carbon dioxide laser affords speed and versatility in terms of depths and angles of approach to an experienced user. Its unique strengths lie with the use of microscopes for a no-touch method of cutting or vaporizing tissue such as performed with craniotomy, microlaryngoscopy or colposcopy.

When used for cutting, the beam is focused at its smallest spot. The depth of the cut is determined by power density and the speed of the incision. The slower the stroke or higher the power density, the deeper will be the cut. To achieve good clean edges on the incision, with minimal charring, traction across the incision line is essential. A mode such as superpulse will give a cleaner incision while decreasing hemostasis.

Incisions made with the carbon dioxide laser heal in much the same way as a conventional wound histologically, though the order of the healing process is slightly different. Scars and wound strength are identical at 20–30 days. In practice, most surgeons see no clinical difference after 7–10 days.

Vaporization of tissue may be performed with a focused or defocused beam (Fig. 14). Although small areas can be vaporized with

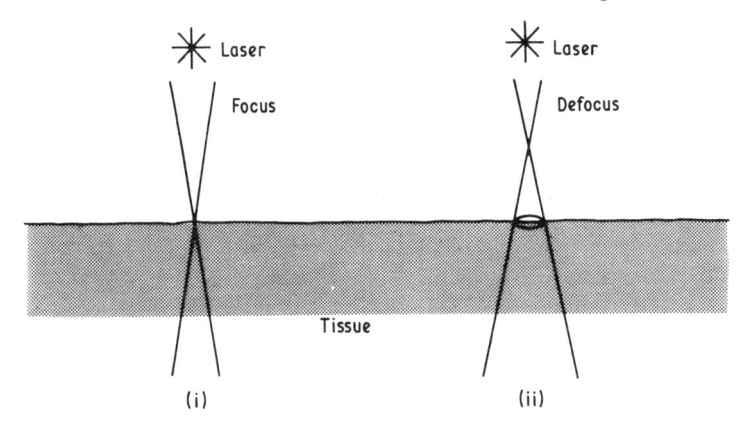

Fig. 14 Focus and defocus. In (i) the laser beam is focused on the tissue in a small spot. In (ii) the laser beam is focused in front of the tissue, so that a defocused spot, of larger area and lower power, impinges on the tissue.

a small spot, larger areas are better handled with a broader spot, and a higher power applied to compensate for the dilution of power density. Pulsing the laser in short bursts allows one to use the maximum power output of the laser to advantage, without the concern for excessive damage.

Even though lasing through char is a classic mistake in using the carbon dioxide laser, one can very precisely remove skin lesions a layer at a time by painting an even layer of black char over the skin, then wiping away this layer with a wet sponge before relasing. Since one does not continue lasing through char, this avoids the high temperatures but it does destroy a very superficial layer of skin that may be wiped away. The cosmetic results can be excellent. When the perfect smoothness of the healed site is not a consideration, more of a stripping technique using higher power densities and faster strokes with blunt spot sizes, will result in precise, superficial vaporization.

The argon laser

The first significant medical use of lasers was the use of argon lasers in the treatment of diabetic retinopathy in 1965. Since then, the extensive experience with argon lasers has resulted in argon laser photocoagulator becoming the treatment of choice for this retinal disorder. Dermatology is another major user of this laser. The laser operates as a sealed tube system with an operating life of only a few years. It is possible to rebuild and recharge these tubes, rather than replacing them with an entirely new tube, at significant savings to the user.

Argon lasers produce a visible blue–green light (488 and 515 nm) which is easily transmitted through clear aqueous tissue. Certain tissue pigment (red or black) as melanin or hemoglobin will absorb the light very effectively. This principle of selective absorption is used to photocoagulate pigmented lesions such as portwine stains (on skin) or endometriosis (intra-abdominally). This light passes through overlying skin, without significant absorption, and reaches the pigmented layer of portwine stains (or other colored lesions) to effect capillary dessication and protein coagulation. Gradual blanching will then begin to occur, perhaps taking many months to fully fade the stain. When the beam is focused to a very small spot and power increased, the power density is high enough to result in cutting or vaporization of tissue.

Many makes and models of ophthalmic lasers are available. Currently, only one make of argon laser is available for general surgical use, which has several different models of various power outputs.

Fiberoptic delivery of the beam is one of the primary advantages of this laser in ophthalmology, dermatology and gynecology.

KTP (Potassium Titanyl Phosphate) laser

Only one company currently produces the KTP laser for medical application. This is an Nd:YAG laser that uses a crystal of KTP at its output to change the color of light from that of the Nd:YAG (1060 nm) to that of the KTP (532 nm — green light). In industry this is commonly referred to as a frequency doubled YAG laser; the only difference here is that all of the residual 1060 nm light has been filtered out to leave only 532 nm. It has nothing in common with the tissue effects of a Nd:YAG laser.

The wavelength is slightly different from that of the argon laser (it has a greener color). This wavelength has a higher specificity for hemoglobin in skin lesions and endometriosis, although clinically their effects are identical (see argon laser tissue effects in Chapter 2). The argon laser produces a continuous wave output of a steady power, where the KTP is a high frequency Q-switched system of around 25 khz. Both produce an average maximum power of around 15 (plus or minus) watts, and both are fiberoptically delivered.

The advantages and disadvantages of each type of system come from comparing the operation of the laser itself, ease of use, types of fiber delivery systems, and safety features. Both types are good lasers for medical use.

The Nd:YAG (Neodymium: Yttrium Aluminum Garnet) laser

The laser that is best suited for primary coagulative properties is the Nd:YAG. When used as a non-contact beam, it coagulates 4–6 mm in depth and with some manipulation will handle vessels up to around 4 mm.

Nd:YAG is a solid crystal which is stimulated to emit near infrared light at 1060 nm. Medical lasers produce 60 to 100 watts of maximum power and are fiberoptically transmitted.

The light is transmitted through clear liquids, which allows its use in the eye or other water-filled cavities such as the bladder or uterus. Its absorption by tissue is not as color-specific as argon, but the darker the tissue, the better the absorption. It is an excellent tool for tissue coagulation in endoscopic applications such as bronchoscopy, cystoscopy and gastroscopy.

Its use with contact probes made from sapphire, diamond or quartz allows both the fine cutting, vaporization, or coagulation of tissue with precision and the avoidance of excessive tissue damage. Synthetic sapphire probes are the most commonly used material for medical use (Chapter 4). This creates an overlap in tissue effects more commonly associated with the carbon dioxide laser. Each has its own advantages.

The dye laser

Several wavelengths of dye lasers are now in medical use. In this laser a suitable organic dye is illuminated with a strong light source, usually the beam of an argon laser or flash lamps, to produce light of various wavelengths. The color of the laser can be controlled by varying the type of dye and the tuning elements in the laser — hence the name **tunable dye lasers**. Dye lasers are generally more sensitive than other medical lasers and are treated appropriately.

It is used where the selective absorption characteristics of the tissue suggest the application of certain colors of laser light. The tunability of this laser is used in ophthalmology to work in different areas of the retina with various colors.

A 577 nm (yellow light) pulsed dye laser is used to great advantage in cosmetic vascular lesions because of the high specificity of hemoglobin to this wavelength. The high peak power, short duration pulse also helps localize thermal damage by applying the beam at a faster rate than heat damage can spread to adjacent tissue. This pulsing technique is important in several laser applications.

A 504 nm pulsed dye laser is used to fragment kidney stones impacted in the ureter or otherwise inaccessible to shock wave lithotripsy. This laser sets up a concussive shock wave on the stone when the fiber is fired in direct contact with it. A similar system is being used experimentally for calcified atherosclerotic plaque.

A continuous wave dye laser, at 630 nm (red light) is used in photodynamic therapy (see Chapter 5). The red light corresponds to a particular absorption peak of a drug such as HpD (hematoporphyrin derivative).

The excimer laser

The excimer constitutes a class of a dozen or so lasers. The term *excimer* is derived from excited dimer and refers to a molecule which is comparatively stable when excited, but which, when it loses energy by emitting a photon, splits up into its component parts. Conditions are therefore ideal for lasing, since this removal of molecules in the resting state results in a population inversion, described earlier. Characteristically, excimer lasers emit in the ultraviolet spectrum, and deliver energies of about 0.1 joules in a pulse duration of around 20 nanoseconds (10^{-9} seconds). Three primary types of excimers are at present in investigational use in medicine.

Of greatest general interest is the 193 nm argon fluoride excimer. This wavelength is transmitted via an articulated arm (like the carbon dioxide laser). Special types of fibers are in development but are not yet practical. It theoretically removes tissue by a nonthermal mechanism of photolysis. Whatever the mechanism, it can achieve a high degree of precision, creating incisions on the cornea with no thermal shrinkage, and achieving predictable depths per pulse in the micron range. It is being examined primarily for corneal work and sees interest in dentistry and orthopedics.

The krypton fluoride laser produces light of 248 nm. However, given the mutagenicity of this wavelength its medical use has been limited.

The xenon chloride laser, producing light at 308 nm, is easily transmitted through conventional fibers and is not mutagenic. It still contains a high energy per pulse, and is being examined most aggressively for cardiovasuclar applications in laser angioplasty.

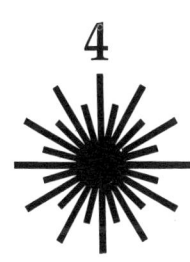

4 Laser Beam Delivery Systems

Much of the development work in laser systems is in the area of delivery devices, i.e. how the light is delivered to the desired target. Delivery devices can create a significant overlap in the effects and applications of the various types of laser systems, remembering that the ultimate laser – tissue interaction mechanism is tissue heating.

Carbon dioxide lasers

At present, an articulated arm is required to deliver the beam to the treatment site. The arm is a hollow tube that has several joints, or articulations, to allow it to be somewhat maneuverable and flexible. The articulations contain reflective mirrors that bounce the beam out through the end regardless of its position. Care must be taken with these arms to avoid jarring impacts which can cause misalignment of the mirrors. Both fixed, and adjustable mirror arms can be knocked out of alignment.

Fibers made of exotic crystals are under development by several companies for carbon dioxide lasers. Conventional quartz fibers will not work. Though the companies should be commended for their development efforts, carbon dioxide laser fibers are not yet practical on a day to day surgical level. Even when good fibers are developed, they are still problematic in causing a loss of the good qualities of a TEM_{00} beam, such as the mode and power. Fibers, when sufficiently developed, will simply be used as attachments to articulated arms in those situations for which endoscopic delivery of carbon dioxide laser is desired.

One company has marketed a hollow waveguide, similar to a fiber, for carbon dioxide laser delivery. This is a slender, hollow tube that propagates the beam via hundreds of glancing internal reflections, until it emerges from the end. This waveguide, called an airfiber, is about 1.5 mm in diameter and somewhat flexible. The power

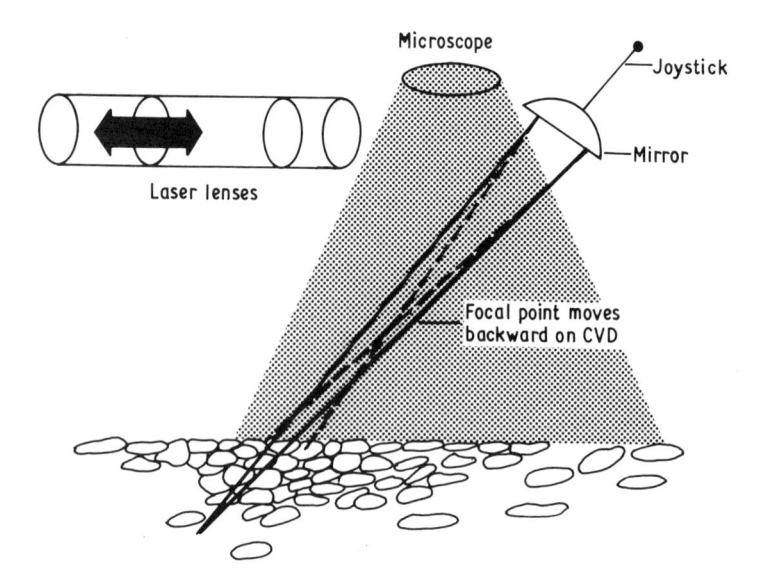

Fig. 15 Micromanipulator.

density is highest within about 1 mm of the waveguide tip, and the spot rapidly increases past that distance.

Various devices are attached to the end of the articulated arm. A **micromanipulator** is used to couple the laser to an operating microscope. A lens system in this manipulator allows the spot size to be

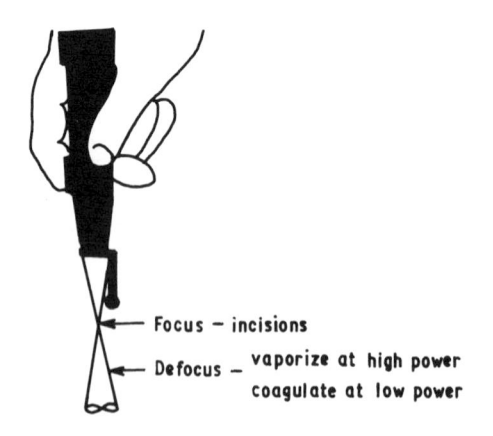

Fig. 16 Use of handpiece.

continuously varied (Fig. 15). A 'joystick' is attached to a reflecting mirror which allows the surgeon to direct the beam. Handpieces allow the freehand use of the laser in the fashion of a laser scalpel, though the weight and resistance of the articulated arm does make it somewhat awkward. The handpiece is simply pulled away from the target to defocus the beam (Fig. 16).

Rigid carbon dioxide laser **bronchoscopes** and **laparoscopes** allow use of the laser down the trachea or into the abdomen respectively. These require special scopes and couplers to direct the laser beam down a straight channel.

Computer-laser scanners are used like an electronic micromanipulator on the microscope. This allows the surgeon to outline any irregular area or shape and automatically lase that pattern. This serves as a convenience item in some situations, but does not expand laser use over that which can be done manually.

Argon and KTP lasers

These are delivered primarily through fiberoptics which may be used as the bare fiber, or terminate into micromanipulators or handpieces. Fiber tips are cooled by either flowing gas around the tip of the fiber (the fiber is enclosed in a sheath for that purpose), or by using the bare fiber within a fluid environment which keeps the tip cool. Fibers are generally 0.6mm or 0.8mm in diameter, but smaller sizes are available. Adding the sheath increases diameters to roughly 1.0–2.0mm.

Fibers, for any laser, are generally used in a non-contact manner. Spot size continuously increases as the fiber is pulled away from the target, causing power density to rapidly fall. Fibers are usually fired about 1–2cm from the target, but this distance can be varied by varying the power output.

Fibers, for most lasers, can also be drawn across tissue, in direct contact with it. The smallest spots and highest power densities are right at the tip, so this will allow the fiber to cut and dissect through tissue. This works best under fluid, to keep the tip cool. This does somewhat abuse the fiber, which will burn out at the tip after a short while, but they can be trimmed and repolished at the tip with minimal effort. These fibers may be delivered through standard flexible or rigid endoscopes and laparascopes.

Opthalmic use of the argon (or krypton, or Q-switched Nd:YAG) laser is almost always through the slit lamp, similar to a micromanipulator on an operating microscope. Some intraoperative argon ophthalmic procedures use slender probes on the end of fibers for intraocular delivery.

Dye lasers

The 504 nm (green) and 577 nm (yellow) which are used for their thermal and/or shock wave effects, are used with small fibers the same way as argon and KTP. The fibers used for lithotripsy (504 nm) are generally much thinner than the standard 0.6 mm argon laser fibers.

The fibers used for photodynamic therapy at 630 nm are used to diffuse the red light uniformly into tissue, rather than concentrating it for thermal effects. The key aspect of the fiber is the type of diffuser used at the tip. Cylinder diffusers shine the light uniformly through the sides of a slender cylinder around the tip. This is used in tubular structures such as the trachea. Light bulb diffusers uniformly spread the light in all directions, as with a light bulb, and are used in structures such as the bladder. Diffusing lenses shine the light evenly onto the skin. Though not used for thermal effects, the interfaces of the fibers and diffusers do accumulate some heat, causing the tips to burn up and lose function after a while.

Excimer lasers

Still in the investigational stage in medicine, most of these wavelengths may be delivered through conventional fibers. The 193 nm argon fluoride, however, does not pass through regular fibers and currently uses articulated arms.

Nd:YAG lasers

These are also fiberoptically delivered lasers, with the exception of the ophthalmic Q-switched Nd:YAG. Standard 0.2 mm to 0.8 mm quartz or glass fibers are either air, or liquid cooled. The sheathed fibers have a total diameter of roughly 1.0–2.0 mm. Because of the higher powers of the Nd:YAG laser compared to the argon or KTP, they have acquired a wider range of applications.

One of the most significant developments in laser delivery systems over the last few years is the sapphire contact probe, used primarily with the Nd:YAG laser – though it could physically function with the argon or KTP.

Sapphire probes, used only at low powers of around 1–20 watts,

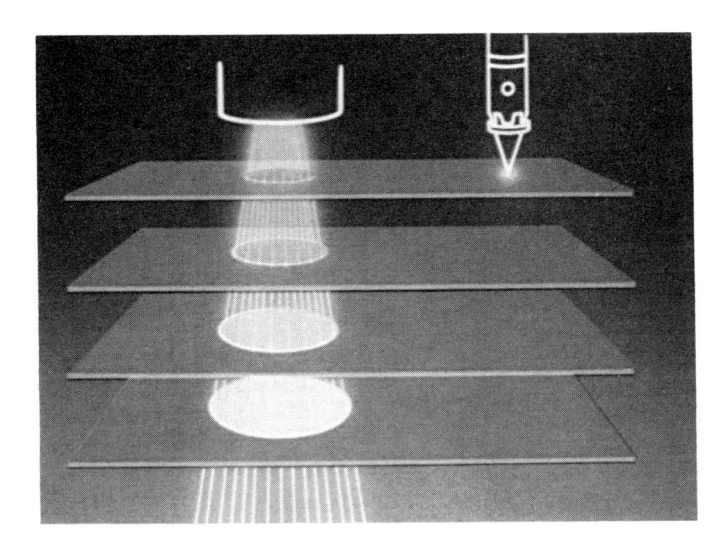

Fig. 17 Divergence of the laser from the non-contact bare fiber (left) compared with the non-divergent SLT contact sapphire probe (right), which produces tissue effects only where it touches.

limit the spread of thermal damage normally associated with the Nd:YAG, and create similar cutting and vaporizing effects as the carbon dioxide laser. Though not a panacea for allowing the Nd:YAG laser to become the universal laser for all applications, these probes do significantly expand the versatility of this laser.

Contact probes, unlike conventional fibers, work only when in direct contact with tissue. This gives tactile stimulation back to the surgeon and allows for a much shorter learning curve. It also means that underlying tissue will not be affected (Figs. 17 and 18), unlike the carbon dioxide laser. Though easier to learn and used in similar procedures to the carbon dioxide laser they do not offer a non-contact approach for more remote access.

These probes work through a combination of concentrating power densities at the small tips and the heating of the crystal sapphire itself. The probe transmits about 35% of the light and 65–70% is converted into heat. Regardless of the exact mechanism of action, they allow for smooth, clean, dry cuts, with lateral tissue damage of only about 0.5–1.0 mm. Various shapes of probes create different effects such as cutting, chiseling, vaporizing or contact coagulation of tissue (Fig. 19).

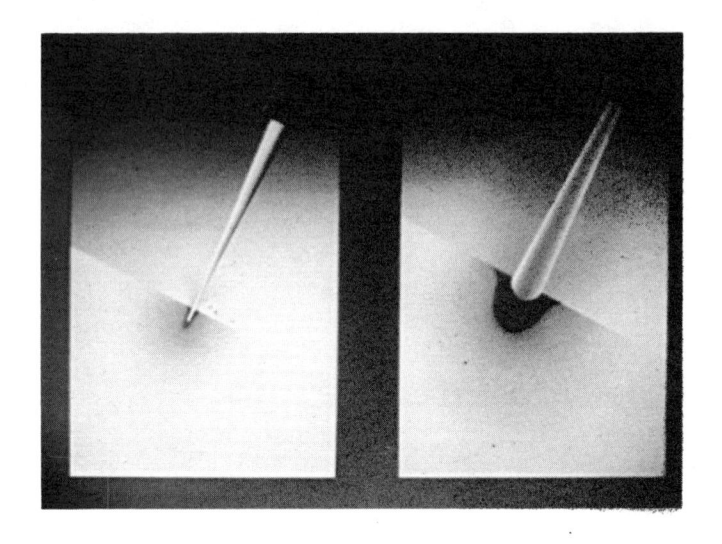

Fig. 18 Contact laser surgery (left) produces minimal lateral tissue damage compared with higher energy non-contact techniques (right).

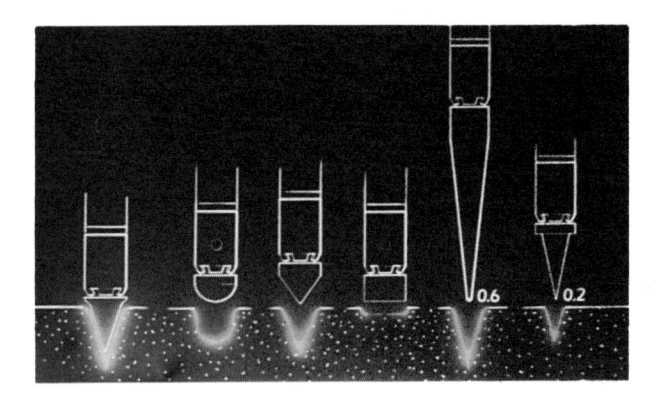

Fig. 19 Geometrical shapes of the SLT contact probes® and their tissue effects at equal power and time.

Photographs by courtesy of Surgical Laser Technologies, One Great Valley Pkwy, Malvern, Pennsylvania, USA.

Probes must be held in contact with tissue when in use, otherwise they will quickly accumulate energy, heat and may be damaged. The fibers for the probes are cooled either by gas or fluid (both through a sheath), and the probe mount should be kept free of tissue accumulation so that the coolant can flow. Fibers with the contact probes have a total diameter of around 1.8 mm or 2.2 mm. They may be used as handheld scalpels, or delivered through flexible or rigid endoscopes on the ends of the fibers.

Micromanipulators are available for some Nd:YAG lasers, but their usefulness is somewhat limited. When used in this non-contact fashion, the Nd:YAG usually causes diffuse coagulation, in contradiction to the objectives of most microscopic procedures. There are exceptions, and the Nd:YAG can always be used with a fiberoptic hand applicator while viewing the field through the microscope.

Aiming beams

Some of the lasers are invisible to the eye, such as the carbon dioxide and Nd:YAG, and use a low power, red, helium neon laser as the guide light. Some Nd:YAG lasers have various colors available as guide lights, and some use a white xenon (non-laser) light.

Visible lasers such as the krypton, argon or KTP usually use the laser on a very low setting as its own guide light. With fiber delivery, or contact probes, one is frequently so close to the target that a guide light may be unnecessary.

5   Overview of Clinical Applications

At this point in time, the medical applications of the laser are so numerous that it is not possible to discuss them all in one chapter of an introductory guide to lasers. We shall, however, cover most of the major, and more established laser procedures currently used.

The advantages of laser surgery vary with each type of procedure, each type of laser and sometimes from case to case. Realizing the full advantage of the laser assumes it is applied appropriately. Conventional techniques will always give better results than a misapplied laser.

Potential **advantages** of various lasers collectively include:

- Dry surgical field
- Reduced blood loss
- Reduced edema
- Limited fibrosis and stenosis
- Fiberoptic delivery
- No interference with monitoring equipment
- Potential reduction in spread of metastasis
- Precision
- Fewer instruments in the field
- Reduced postoperative pain (selectively)
- Sterilization of the impact site
- Contact or no-touch technique as an option

The carbon dioxide laser is still the most commonly used laser in an operating room setting. It has widespread applications that make use of its cutting and vaporizing abilities. Its secondary cautery effects are also helpful.

The argon laser is the most prevalent overall, though not in an operating room setting. Its primary use has been in ophthalmology as a retinal photocoagulator. It is also widely used for colored skin lesions in dermatology and is beginning to see greater endoscopic use.

The Nd:YAG laser is the fastest growing segment for laser surgery in an operating room setting. Its fiberoptic delivery, high power when needed, and now the contact probes for fine cutting and vaporizing, makes this a very versatile instrument in many specialties. General surgery, which sees little laser use otherwise, may develop significant use for contact Nd:YAG laser surgery. The Nd:YAG's use in ophthalmology as a Q-switched device has seen explosive growth over the last few years.

An overview of the major specialties that have current laser use is as follows.

Gynecology

This specialty probably has the largest potential volume of uses for the carbon dioxide laser. It is used in colposcopy, laparoscopy for endometriosis, and laparotomy for infertility work.

The use of argon, KTP, and Nd:YAG lasers is also seeing significant use in gynecology. Previous chapters discuss how each system may be manipulated to cut, vaporize, or coagulate tissue.

In laparoscopy the laser provides a significant advantage in providing a method to treat mild to moderate endometriosis at the time of the diagnostic look. It can vaporize or coagulate endometriomas and dissect adhesions. It is good for clearing obstructed tubes and ovaries and can totally eliminate abdominal bleeding. The carbon dioxide laser has, until now, been the primary instrument for laparoscopy. The articulated arm and need for a laser coupling cube has been awkward, and smoke production creates the need for continuous high flow insufflation to clear the smoke and maintain pneumoperitoneum. Fiberoptic laser systems are the definite trend in laser laparoscopy because they are easier to work with and eliminate much of the smoke. These include the argon, KTP and Nd:YAG (particularly with contact probes) lasers.

Abdominal cysts and tumors may be excised or vaporized with similar benefits. The ability to vaporize tissue with minimal surrounding damage, even when associated with dense and extensive tissue adhesions, has proven of great value for patients with complications of pelvic inflammatory disease.

The carbon dioxide laser is used in microtuboplasty to cut the tube prior to reanastomis. The benefits of this are more controversial but it does eliminate bleeding. A laser incision also provides a precise, atraumatic means of opening the end of a closed tube in a bloodless fashion. In neosalpingotomy, the power density is lowered and the laser used to 'paint' a ring around the end of the tube. The shrinkage causes a flowering of the tube. When extensive adhesions are encountered, particularly in the cul-de-sac on the bowel, laser can reduce operative time by one-third to one-half.

Uterine myomas may be removed by vaporization or excision. A microlaser myomectomy provides hemostasis and precision when removing fibroids.

Laser has been used in cornual reimplantation. Radical procedures, such as radical vulvectomies, and excision of large vascular tumors are performed with laser for better hemostasis. These applications require higher power from a carbon dioxide laser (50–60 watts), or contact probes on a Nd:YAG laser.

One of the most common uses of the carbon dioxide laser is the treatment of cervical intraepithelial neoplasia (CIN) for either ablation or excision. This is most commonly done through the colposcope. The Nd:YAG laser with contact probes, or green light, will perform an adequate excision or ablation, but may be slower than the carbon dioxide laser. The carbon dioxide laser is thought by some to be the primary laser for this application.

Laser vaporization of the cervix provides advantages over cauterization, knife conization or cryotherapy. It leaves the cervix in a more viable condition, with no stenosis and minimal scarring. It is possible to tailor the treatment to the extent of the disease thus ensuring that the entire diseased area has been treated. It eliminates the heavy discharge associated with cryosurgery and is significantly more precise. Laser colposcopy is an outpatient or office procedure for ablations — a significant advantage. Similar advantages are gained in the laser treatment of vaginal intraepithelial neoplasia (VIN).

Genital warts such as condyloma accuminata may be treated to advantage with the laser. The carbon dioxide laser not only vaporizes the lesions (frequently through the colposcope) but can also flash sterilize the skin between lesions. This kills the latent virus and reduces frequency and extent of recurrence. Argon or KTP lasers may be used for superficial lesions through the colposcope. Contact probes on the Nd:YAG are used to superficially vaporize the warts in a contact fashion.

Laser hysteroscopy is beginning to develop. Uterine septae may be cut with contact probes on the Nd:YAG, or bare fibers with the argon, KTP, or Nd:YAG lasers. The main use of the Nd:YAG in hysteroscopy is in endometrial ablation as a treatment for chronic menorrhagia. The procedure, which may be performed on a same-day-surgery basis, uses the laser to 'cook' the endometrium, creating a type of Asherman's syndrome of scarring of the uterus. Not all women become totally amenorheic after treatment, but almost all are happy with results. Retreatment is possible if desired. The contact Nd:YAG has also been used for the laparoscopic outpatient treatment of ectopic tubal pregnancies.

Otorhinolaryngology

This is one of the developed uses for the carbon dioxide laser endoscopically because of the no-touch technique, long reach of the laser, absence of postoperative swelling or stenosis, dry operative field, and greatly reduced postoperative pain.

Application of the carbon dioxide laser to laryngeal diseases requiring microlaryngoscopy has provided a degree of precision otherwise impossible. Although the carbon dioxide laser is predominantly used in otorhinolaryngology, the green laser (argon or KTP) may also be used through a micromanipulator to achieve this same no-touch precision. The precision cutting and excellent healing with each laser is more advantageous than its hemostasis. Postoperative pain is minimal and most procedures may be done on a same-day surgery basis. The need for tracheotomy is reduced. These cases require general anesthesia and appropriate safety precautions must be taken because of the flammability of the endotracheal tube.

Surgical applications of the laser in microlaryngoscopy include vocal cord nodules, polyps, hyperkeratosis, granulomas, arytenoidectomy, Quincke's edema, cysts, webs and laryngeal stenosis.

The treatment of congenital and acquired lesions in pediatric surgery has proven the carbon dioxide laser to be a remarkably effective tool. Airway lesions are more critical in the child than the adult because of the size of the airway, making the laser ideal for infants. Its properties of hemostasis, enhanced visibility, lack of postoperative edema and scarring, all contribute to its successful application in pediatrics.

Recurrent respiratory papillomatosis occurs throughout the anterior nasal cavity, subglottis and mainstem bronchi. These relatively inaccessible locations make the carbon dioxide laser ideal for the removal of all visible papillomas by vaporization. Complete hemostasis allows all visible lesions to be destroyed under constant visual control. There is minimal damage to underlying tissue and the airway can be maintained so that tracheotomy is usually unnecessary. Recurrences are not eliminated, but a large percentage of patients go into a year or more of remission after two or more excisions with the laser.

The carbon dioxide laser has been used for intranasal work such as turbinectomy, choanal atresia, and telangiectasia. Contact probes on the Nd:YAG laser may actually work better than the carbon dioxide for most intranasal cutting and vaporizing because of the vascularity. Laser has also been used effectively to treat rhinophyma, polyposis, synechia and granuloma.

Laser tonsillectomy is most appropriately carried out in patients with coagulopathies such as hemophilia. Proponents of laser tonsillectomy on normal patients point out improved hemostasis and reduced postoperative pain.

Lesions of the oral cavity, such as leukoplakia and other benign lesions, may be excised or vaporized. Tongue releases may also be performed with the laser.

Argon and KTP lasers have been used successfully in otology for stapedotomy because of their small spot size. The laser punches a series of holes in the footplate of the stapes that allow an area to be tapped out (like a postage stamp) with minimal mechanical trauma to middle and inner ear structures. The prosthetic piston will be placed in this hole. The carbon dioxide laser has also begun to see use in this application, the primary difference being that it is fast-pulsed to create one small round hole into which the piston is inserted. A fast pulse in the superpulse mode, with the laser finely focused, helps create the smallest hole (around 0.5mm). Most medical carbon dioxide lasers are capable of being manipulated to this degree of precision. Lasers have also been used for tympanoplasty, myringotomy, treatment of fixed malleus syndrome, and removal of growths, though most are not well accepted laser procedures.

The contact YAG laser has been successfully used in excising lesions of the tongue, including a hemiglossectomy with virtually no bleeding and little pain. Similar applications are in major head and neck surgery including thyroidectomy.

Pulmonary medicine

Tumors of the trachea and bronchi may be palliated with the carbon dioxide or Nd:YAG lasers.

The carbon dioxide laser is precise, somewhat hemostatic and immediately vaporizes the obstruction. A rigid carbon dioxide laser bronchoscope and coupler cube are required for delivery of the beam. The long focal length of the laser lens also allows the beam to remain in focus over a long distance. This is a potential hazard and one must carefully avoid penetrating the trachea and underlying great vessels.

The Nd:YAG laser is also used to treat airway obstructions even more effectively than with the carbon dioxide laser. The Nd:YAG can be used with the bare fiber to achieve coagulation and the necrotic tissue debrided through the scope. Contact probes may be used to more finely chisel and vaporize a lumen through the tumor. A combination of these techniques may be necessary.

A flexible bronchoscope may be used with the Nd:YAG fiber for access to bronchi beyond the carina, though when the tumor is more accessible, a rigid scope is preferred because of the ability to debride tissue better, the greater suction and finer manipulation at the tip of the scope. A special rigid bronchoscope is available from several companies that has been modified for Nd:YAG laser use by swiveling the proximal port and providing channels for fibers.

Ordinarily one must be very conscious of the deep coagulation that the non-contact Nd:YAG can achieve. Powers are frequently limited to around 25 watts for 0.5 seconds, for safety reasons, since most tumors would be overlying the carina or large vessels around bronchi. The coagulation could extend into the underlying vessel, causing necrosis and perforation within one or two days. A good visualization of the anatomy and use of lower power helps prevent this. Contact probes limit the damage to about 0.5 mm. Tumors that occupy the mid portion of the trachea may be handled more aggressively. Extraluminal tumors that compress the airway cannot be treated with either the carbon dioxide or Nd:YAG lasers by bronchoscopy.

Neurosurgery

The primary instrument in neurosurgery has remained the carbon dioxide laser, for the same reasons as for microlaryngoscopy. The carbon dioxide laser is an ideal instrument for microscopic use, long reach into small holes, and precision.

The Nd:YAG is a very useful adjunctive type of laser for this field. It has been helpful in shriveling very vascular tumors, and has begun to be used in treating certain aneurysms and arteriovenous malformation (AVMs). Contact probes on handpieces, used while viewing through the microscope, offer a more precise way to use the Nd:YAG for closing down small feeder vessels.

Most craniotomies may be made small when performing laser surgery. An orange sized tumor could be removed through a quarter size opening by coring the center of the mass. Fewer instruments are in the field of view and this, coupled with the good hemostasis, makes it much easier to see the anatomy. In debulking techniques of large bloody tumors it offers an atraumatic, no-touch instrument, reasonable hemostasis and good visibility. The no-touch technique with the carbon dioxide laser is of significant advantage here. The less pulling, tugging and manipulation of tissue that is done the better the patient's postoperative recovery. According to many neurosurgeons, laser-treated patients are more likely to be alert, up and around the day after surgery.

Meningiomas which have tough dural attachments may be easily 'peeled away' with a laser. Their use for acoustic neuromas has become a standard due to their precision and preservation of the acoustic nerve. Lasers are similarly ideal to preserve function when treating tumors around the optic chiasm and nerve. Low power, short pulses help to eliminate heat spread into the nerves. Tumor remnants may be shaved one cell layer at a time from arteries, with no damage to the underlying vessel. Correct technique is critical here. The Nd:YAG laser, when used in a non-contact manner to dessicate and coagulate large tumors, causes it to pucker and peel away from normal brain tissue.

In transphenoidal hypophysectomy, the carbon dioxide laser offers an atraumatic, no-touch technique that eliminates instruments in the narrow canal of the speculum. Soft pituitary tumors can be removed by suction and do not require use of a laser. Recurrent adenomas, particularly those that have been treated with radiation therapy, are hard and rubbery, and very difficult to remove. The laser is ideal for this purpose.

Spinal tumors also benefit from laser surgery, particularly intramedullary tumors. Manipulation of the cord is kept to a minimum, resulting in less damage to both cord and nerve roots. Lasers may be used for fenestration of syringomyelia to offer a permanent fluid pathway. Intractable pain has been treated with laser lesions of the dorsal root entry zone (DREZ), a more precise and controlled method than other techniques.

The carbon dioxide laser has been used to dissect away back muscle for spinal surgery and laser diskectomy. Both applications are less established although they certainly exhibit no undue risks or complications. The argument for dissecting muscle is that the patient does not experience spasm, as occurs with electrocautery. Postoperative back pain is also markedly reduced. The Nd:YAG laser with contact probes, though slightly slower, can more easily achieve a nice, clean dissection of muscle with better hemostasis.

The laser is also used to remove fractured disks by vaporization while compressing the vertebrae in a continuous fashion to feed the cartilage into the beam. Ordinarily the cartilage is pulled from the intervertebral space in different pieces.

Newer areas include the use of flexible and rigid endoscopes (encephaloscopes) for laser energy delivery, allowing less invasive surgery.

Dermatology and plastic surgery

The carbon dioxide and argon lasers are used extensively in dermatology. The KTP has the same applications as the argon. The Nd:YAG is beginning to see investigational use and may be very good for cavernous types of hemangiomas and keloid revisions.

The pulsed dye laser, at 577 nm (yellow), is starting to be used as a very selective photocoagulator. The wavelength, coupled with short pulse widths, achieves precise vascular coagulation which is beyond the abilities of the continuous wave of the argon.

The argon laser, because of its color selectivity, is used to photo-coagulate pigmented cutaneous lesions such as portwine stains, capillary hemangiomas, telangiectasia, strawberry marks, Campbell DeMorgan senile angiomas, and acne rosacea. It may be used to remove tattoos, treat pyogenic granuloma, sebaceous nevi and the Peutz–Jegher syndrome. Less established uses include keloid scars, subcutaneous varicose veins, road skid burns, moles, warts and nevi of the Osler–Weber–Rendu syndrome. The KTP laser may be used for the same purposes as the argon laser.

Portwine hemangiomas involve an increase in the number of vessels in the subepidermal zone. Lasers, except for the carbon dioxide, transmit through the epidermis as if through a window pane, and coagulate vessels within the dermis. The treatment is performed as a series of applications over several months, resulting in gradual fading. Test areas are first performed to determine which laser, and parameters, provide the best cosmetic result.

Tattoos may be removed with the laser which provides good, but not perfect results. Visible lasers selectively obliterate the dye in a tattoo. Green argon or KTP is used for black and red dyes, and red krypton works with blue or green dyes. Professional tattoos are easier to remove than amateur ones because of the consistency in dye depth. The visible lasers shine through the epidermis, leaving no surface scar. Hypertrophic scarring may be a problem and though the tattoo can be erased, a scar may be left in its image.

The advantage of the carbon dioxide laser in removing tattoos is that it gives uniform vaporization independent of dye color or shape. Although a superficial scar is left, it can be blended at the edges so that no tattoo image remains. It is important not to relase through char, as this could cause significant scarring.

Recently, tattoos have been successfully removed with the Nd:YAG laser. Low levels of Nd:YAG light have been shown to decrease collagen production in fibroblast cultures. This has implications for both reduced scarring, and for the possible excision and treatment of keloids, having in fact been successfully used for this purpose in keloids that were refractory to steroid injection and excision.

All types of surgical lasers produce a sterile field. This is excellent in guarding against sepsis. The laser seals lymphatics, so it is of potential benefit in treatment of cutaneous malignancies.

The carbon dioxide laser has been used in breast surgery to reduce blood loss. Skin incisions made with the carbon dioxide laser produce scars that are cosmetically similar to that of a cold knife.

The scalpel contact probes for the Nd:YAG laser are excellent for use in breast surgery. The skin incision may be made with a knife, and the rest of the dissection performed with the contact Nd:YAG laser. Hemostasis is excellent, with minimal spread of tissue damage, less bleeding, reduced pain and postoperative drainage.

Contact probes are also excellent for raising skin flaps. The dissections are very clean, with no charring, and exceptionally dry. Carbon dioxide lasers may be used as well, but they are more difficult to control to avoid penetrating the flap.

Gastroenterology

Both argon and Nd:YAG lasers have been used endoscopically in the treatment of gastrointestinal disease, the Nd:YAG being the primary treatment modality.

The laser may be used in the endoscopic treatment of bleeding from peptic ulcers. Hemostasis may be achieved by using the laser fiber either in a contact (with probes) or non-contact fashion. In cases which are actively bleeding at the time of endoscopy, and are situated in an area that is difficult to access for contact or heater probes, the laser offers the advantage of being able to coagulate without touching. A jet of coaxial carbon dioxide gas is delivered down the fiber sheath to cool the tip and clear blood from the field of view. The high flow rates of the gas can cause problems in managing the overdistension which is created. Contact Nd:YAG lasers allow the use of coaxial fluid through the sheath of the fiber to keep it cool, which eliminates the distension problems.

Contact probes may be used to coagulate GI bleeders, requiring at least 75% less power, and offering the advantage of mechanical pressure to coapt the vessel walls as it is heated.

Angiomata of the GI tract also respond well to laser, but are of lesser value for the more diffuse lesions, such as hemorrhagic esophagitis, gastritis, or duodenitis. Lasers have little use in the difficult treatment of esophageal varices.

Recanalization of advanced, obstructive tumors is an excellent use of the Nd:YAG laser as a palliative measure. It can provide relief of symptoms, particularly for the dysphagia associated with advanced esophageal and other tumors, unsuitable for other forms of treatment. Obstructions may be coagulated in a non contact fashion, then debrided. Care must be taken at the anterior wall, because of the deep Nd:YAG scatter, to avoid trachealesophageal fistulas.

Obstructions may also be opened with the use of contact vaporizing probes with coaxial water . Limited lateral thermal necrosis decreases the concern for fistulas, but probes should be used parallel to the true lumen. Guidewire and dilation are used to assist the recanalization.

Hemorrhoids have been treated very successfully with both carbon dioxide and Nd:YAG lasers. The carbon dioxide is used primarily for externals and skin tags, and the Nd:YAG for coagulating feeders to the internal veins. Contact probes in the Nd:YAG may be advantageous here in performing a formal hemorrhoidectomy. Techniques vary widely.

Urology

The Nd:YAG laser is the primary instrument for endoscopic procedures, and the carbon dioxide laser for external lesions. Argon or KTP may be used endoscopically and are useful for very superficial bladder tumors.

Similar to gynecologic applications, the carbon dioxide laser can vaporize and sterilize condylomata and external lesions. Partial nephrectomy may be performed with the carbon dioxide laser or contact Nd:YAG laser to significantly reduce blood loss and retain maximum function in the remaining portion of the kidney. One of the developmental uses for low power density carbon dioxide laser is in tissue welding with reanastomosis of the vas deferens.

Urethral strictures have been successfully treated with both argon and Nd:YAG lasers. The contact probe with the Nd:YAG laser is an excellent approach to treatment of strictures as experience has been acquired.

The primary use of the Nd:YAG laser in urology has been the transurethral treatment of multiple, superficial bladder tumors. The laser fiber is passed through the cystoscope with a fiber deflector on the bridge. It is passed into the bladder while instilling with water. The laser causes a homogenous band of necrosis in the mucous membrane of the bladder down to the serosa without seriously compromising the mechanical stability of the bladder wall or causing perforations. The photocoagulation is either contactless or used with the contact probes, bloodless, and interrupts lymphatic drainage. Transurethral catheter drainage of the bladder is eliminated and the procedure itself does not take long to perform. Some procedures are being performed in an office setting.

Tumors up to 2 cm or so may be totally eliminated by the laser while larger ones may be removed via a cutting loop and the tumor bed then laser coagulated. Second sessions for larger tumors are necessary. The laser is especially useful for small, multifocal bladder tumors.

The Nd:YAG laser has been used clinically to treat bladder tumors, penile carcinoma, urethral strictures and prostate cancer. Prostatectomy with laser is still investigational and not yet commonly performed. It is mechanically difficult and a very slow procedure.

A pulsed dye laser producing green light at 504 nm is now being used to fragment kidney stones. A transurethral approach is necessary and a very slender fiber is advanced until it abutts up to the stone. The fiber is sometimes advanced through the sheath of a wire basket, which holds the stone during the procedure. The laser impact develops a type of shock wave that mechanically disintegrates the stone. It works on impacted stones, and those within the pelvis — areas that are more difficult for extracorporeal shock wave lithotripsy (ESWL) to treat.

Oral surgery and dentistry

Laser work in these fields is primarily divided into soft tissue such as the gums, and hard tissue such as enamel and dentin.

The carbon dioxide laser is being used clinically to perform gingivectomy. It has been particularly useful in treating patients with dilantin hyperplasia of the gums because it reduces or eliminates bleeding, sterilizes as it vaporizes, and results in significantly less postoperative pain than conventional techniques. Additionally, the spot may be defocused to vaporize and sculpt areas of gum rather than just incise. One must be careful not to mark underlying teeth with the laser however, and an osteal retractor placed between gum and teeth may serve as an adequate backstop. The contact probe on the Nd:YAG laser has been shown to incise soft tissue without marking the underlying enamel and is replacing the CO_2 laser in this area.

Carbon dioxide lasers have also been used to vaporize dental caries, and to sculpt enamel in preparation for an amalgam (filling). This is a developing area of dental laser use. Appropriate techniques consider the heat buildup of the laser to avoid damage to the pulp, by pulsing and irrigation.

General surgery

This area has sometimes been referred to as the sleeping giant of laser use. More procedures are now carried out with the laser, mostly tumor resections but rapidly expanding into more conventional areas. Most of the work to date has been with carbon dioxide lasers, and the Nd:YAG is just coming into play. The use of contact Nd:YAG laser is significantly expanding laser use into general surgery as a handheld modality that can cut, vaporize, and coagulate tissue.

The laser has been used in the excision, or spot vaporization, of metastases of the liver including anatomical and non-anatomical hepatic resections and in performing partial pancreatectomy and other vascular organ work. A carbon dioxide laser requires fairly high power, 50–60 watts, to work in these vascular areas. Nd:YAG contact probes still require the usual 10–20 watts.

The carbon dioxide laser sterilizes as it vaporizes in a no-touch fashion so it is a good tool to use for debridement of external ulcers. It may also be used in burn debridement to achieve sterility and hemostasis, although the contact Nd:YAG may be technically easier to use here.

Contact YAG laser surgery is finding increasing applications in breast surgery, gall bladder, hernia, thyroid and hemorrhoid operations. Advantages appear to be less bleeding and postoperative pain, with earlier mobilization.

Orthopedics

Orthopedic surgeons have very limited uses for the laser at present but much development work is being carried out. The carbon dioxide laser has been used both with a handpiece and through the microscope to vaporize polymethylmethacrylate in the shaft of the femur when replacing artificial joints. Irrigation is necessary to avoid flaming, and high smoke evacuation eliminates the noxious fumes. The laser is best used to core the glue, leaving only a thin crust to chisel out.

Both the carbon dioxide and Nd:YAG lasers have been investigated in arthroscopy. The carbon dioxide laser can operate, but is awkward to use because it will not work in a fluid. The Nd:YAG is also problematic in that it cannot produce the necessary cutting effects. However, recent work with Nd:YAG and sapphire probes has produced encouraging results in knee and shoulder arthoscopic surgery.

The contact scalpel can be used to incise muscle in artificial joint replacement and spinal surgery.

An exciting prospect for reconstructive orthopedic microsurgery is the use of laser to achieve tissue welding. This has been done with low power density carbon dioxide lasers, and with argon lasers. A 1.3 micron Nd:YAG laser, with programmed dosimetry, has investigational approval for laser fusion on several types of tissue. Best results have so far been shown on vessels and nerves.

Ophthalmology

Ophthalmologists were the pioneers of lasers in surgery. Lasers have been used for precise photocoagulation of the retina since the mid-1960s. The argon laser is the primary photocoagulator. Krypton lasers, with their yellow and red wavelengths, are also used by retinal specialists to achieve greater control in the macular area. Q-switch, and to a lesser degree mode-locked, Nd:YAG lasers see heavy use in ophthalmology. All these lasers may be used as standalone units, or commonly the argon and krypton are combined in one unit and delivered through the same slit lamp. Some companies also allow mating of their Q-switched Nd:YAG into the argon/krypton slit lamp. The tubes on the argon and krypton lasers may be refurbished rather than purchasing whole new tubes.

The use of the carbon dioxide laser has been very minimal. As a vaporizing instrument it has been used to excise scleral tumors. It

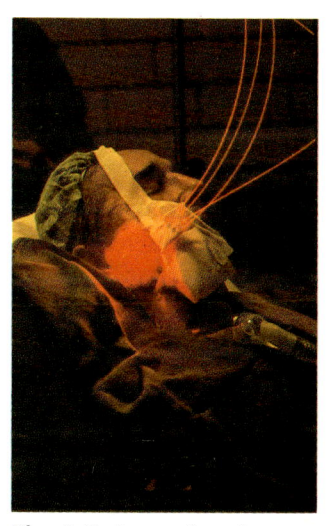

Plate I Patient undergoing photoradiation therapy with a dye laser for a tumor in his right cheek. Four fibers are delivering laser light which can be seen shining through the skin.

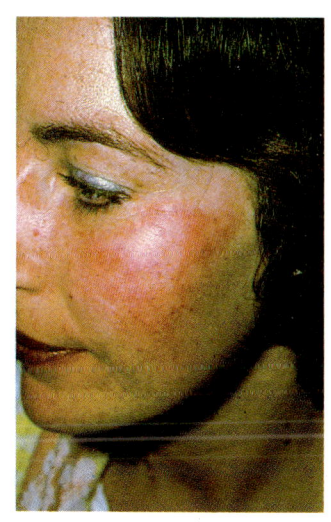

Plate II(a) Patient with a portwine stain (birthmark) on her cheek.

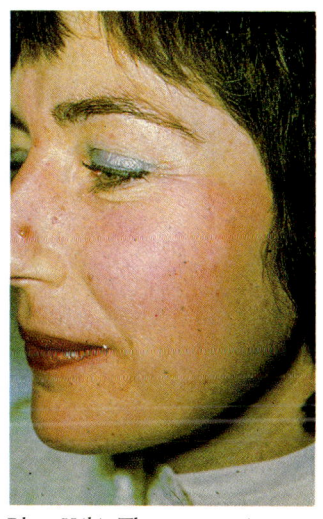

Plate II(b) The same patient after treatment with an argon laser, showing the greatly improved cosmetic appearance which can be achieved.

(Photographs by courtesy of Mr J.A.S. Carruth, Royal South Hants Hospital, Southampton).

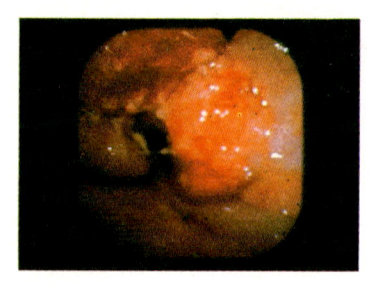

Plate III(a) Tumor of the esophagus. The tumor is the bright red mass in center, and has almost completely blocked the esophagus leaving only a very small opening (the black area to the left of the tumor).

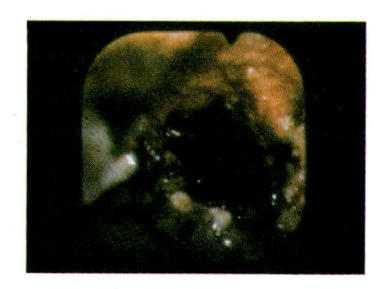

Plate III(b) The tumor has been removed by treatment with a Nd:YAG laser thereby clearing the blockage.

(Photographs by courtesy of Dr S.G. Bown, University College Hospital, London, and first published in *The Proceedings of the Royal Institution of Great Britain*, 55, 177–97, 1983).

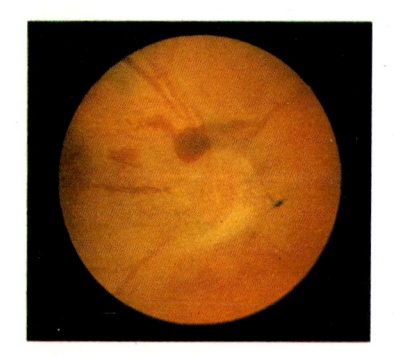

Plate IV(a) Proliferative diabetic retinopathy in an insulin-dependent diabetic patient of 20 years duration. Several areas of hemorrhage with optic disc neovascularization (new vessels) can be seen.

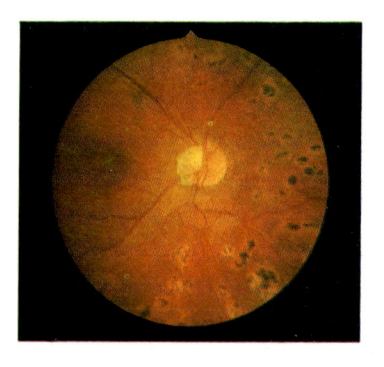

Plate IV(b) Complete regression of the hemorrhage and new vessels has been achieved by pan retinal photocoagulation with an argon laser.

(Photographs by courtesy of Mr R.J. Cooling, Moorfields Eye Hospital, London).

has also been used to create bloodless scleral flaps. The 10,600 nm wavelength cannot be transmitted into the eye as can the argon and Nd:YAG, so it can only be used for open procedures. It has been used in the past through intraocular probes containing infrared windows at the tip, to cut vitreal strands, vaporize small tumors and weld detached retinas, but this laser is rarely if ever used for this anymore.

Argon is the common ophthalmic laser, either used in an office or clinic setting through the slit lamp, or intraoperatively with intraocular probes. Patients with diabetic retinopathy suffer from a proliferation of blood vessels on the retina which are fragile, tend to bleed, and may even tear the retina because of retraction of the vitreous. Panretinal photocoagulation (PRP) with the argon laser may slow or stop progression of the disease, but cannot restore vision already lost, at least in most situations. Numerous lesions are placed on the periphery of the retina to stop proliferation of the vessels. The pigment seeking qualities of the beam causes absorption in the pigment epithelium and the photoreceptor area. A green-only option on the argon allows deeper penetration of the beam with less damage to surface retinal vessels.

The exact mechanism of the induced changes in the retinal microcirculation are not clear. The general principle is that oxygen tension levels are changed so that new vessels do not have to constantly develop. This also provides better oxygenation in the remaining photoreceptors which can actually improve vision in some cases.

Krypton lasers produce yellow and red light. For work in the macular area this light will spare the macula lutea and be absorbed in the pigment epithelium. The yellow xanthophyll pigment is contained in the macula and will not absorb yellow light at all and red light very poorly. Red light is used in treatment of subretinal neovascular membranes. It spares surface vessels and the macula, and destroys the pathological subretinal blood supply. Some types of senile macular degeneration (SMD) are very responsive to laser treatment.

Lasers have also been used in different ways to treat glaucoma. In closed angle glaucoma, iridotomy may be performed with the laser to open a channel for fluid flow between the anterior and posterior chambers. Argon lasers are used for this, but an iris that is blue or light colored does not absorb the light as readily as a dark one. Using the argon to cauterize a spot on the iris, then performing the iridotomy with a Q-switched Nd:YAG, seems to work easier on these light colored eyes. Laser iridotomy has a problem with long term patency, but it is a simple procedure that may be quickly and easily repeated. The surgical alternative to laser iridotomy is iridectomy. This invasive surgical procedure requires operating room time and facilities. Even with laser treatment, medication will probably still be required to control intraocular pressures.

Argon laser trabeculoplasty is used to treat open angle glaucoma. The laser creates multiple lesions around the periphery of the iris into the trabecular meshwork. It thermally shrinks the mesh, creating larger spaces for fluid to flow through. The contact lens that is used for treatment has an angled mirror around the edge to bounce the light into the meshwork. Patients can usually maintain acceptable introcular pressures with minimal medication.

Never developments include the use of the contact probes with the continuous wave YAG laser in performing occuloplastic surgery, treatment of glaucoma and retinal applications.

Pulsed Nd:YAG lasers, of the Q-switched or mode locked variety, produce nonlinear effects at a small focal point. Tremendous peak powers in the millions of watts delivered in an ultrashort burst cause a tiny concussive effect at the 50 micron spot. One can see the spark and listen to the crack as it literally snaps apart a membrane. The intense focus of the laser pulse creates an ionization effect on the target and works by sonic, or acoustical means — a little sonic boom. This is a cold cutting effect sometimes called **photodisruption**, and the lasers are called photodisruptors. The ionized plasma — the spark — absorbs the laser light and forms a shield which protects the retina from the beam. The large cone angle of focus also helps protect the retina.

The primary use of photodisruptors is secondary to cataract surgery, for posterior capsulotomy. They are also used for vitreoretinal and glaucoma surgery, and to cut internal sutures.

In posterior capsulotomy, the laser is not actually used to remove the primary cataract. However, on cataracts suspected of being very hard, the surgeon sometimes will crack apart the hard lens in the clinic with the laser before taking them to surgery for conventional surgery. This makes it easier to remove a hard cataract. When the diseased lens is removed, the posterior capsule is left intact to provide support for the intraocular lens implant (IOL) and decrease the likelihood of some postoperative complications. Unfortunately, this membrane later becomes clouded in a large percentage of these patients. Without laser, an invasive surgical procedure is required to open the clouded membrane. Instead, the laser snaps an opening in the membrane in just a few minutes with several laser shots.

When a photodisrupting laser is used for procedures that may involve a blood supply, such as cutting vitreal strands, an argon laser should be available. If the cold cut of the Nd:YAG creates a small intraocular hemorrage it is important to be able to cauterize it immediately with the argon. Some ophthalmic Nd:YAG lasers have what is termed a 'free running' or thermal mode. This allows continuous wave operation for photocoagulation. The power is not sufficient to use this mode in other surgical specialties that use continuous wave Nd:YAG lasers.

Developmentally, there is considerable excitement over the use of the excimer laser, in particular the 193 nm argon fluoride, for use in corneal work. The very fine non-thermal cut is consistent and predictable on the micron level. It could theoretically even be used for corneal sculpting. It is being examined to take corneal buttons and perform radial keratotomy. One device under commercial development will use the scanning properties of the HeNe laser to sense the shape of the cornea, and the excimer laser will be used with computer control to recontour it to correct vision.

Vascular surgery

Laser work in this area centers primarily around laser recanalization to open closed vessels or tissue welding. Work is being done in this area with just about every type of laser imaginable. It is impossible to predict just which type of laser or delivery system will ultimately prove superior, but some of the major approaches will be discussed.

Tissue welding of small vessels is occurring experimentally in laboratories and has been used clinically in a few cases. Low power density carbon dioxide lasers are pulsed on the seam to create an immediate and permanent laser weld with power densities in the broad range of 5–80 watts/cm^2. One way to achieve steady, low power density is to use a milliwatt output laser. This produces a very stable output which may be focused to microspot sizes and still retain a sufficiently low power density. This has worked best for carbon dioxide lasers. It is also possible to use low power (0.5–3.0 watts) from a conventional carbon dioxide laser and simply broaden the spot sufficiently to achieve very low power density. Some regular surgical carbon dioxide lasers have milliwatt capability. Normal output carbon dioxide laser tubes are not very stable at very low milliwatt powers and this is not an optimum solution. It is possible to use an attenuator delivery system for a regular carbon dioxide laser and achieve stable milliwatt powers.

Argon lasers used with handheld fibers at 0.5–3.0 watts output may be used to weld arteriotomies with good results. Argon has also been used to achieve vessel fusion. A 1.3 micron Nd:YAG laser, programmed for the correct dosimetry on various tissues, is also being investigated as a better alternative to the carbon dioxide laser for tissue fusion. The contact Nd:YAG has also been used in these areas.

Laser recanalization of blood vessels is a major topic in laser medicine. Fibers are passed through endoscopes or catheters into the vessel and used to open the blockage. The type of laser used and its delivery system are two separate areas of development. Argon, Nd:YAG and excimer lasers are the frontrunners for the wavelength. Delivery systems used include bare fibers, hot metal tips, sapphire probes, 'ball tip' fibers, quartz domed fibers including multichannel bundles, and handheld needle delivery systems for carbon dioxide lasers as an intraoperative approach.

The hot metal tips are used with the argon and Nd:YAG lasers as the heat input. These bullet shaped tips come in a variety of configurations to provide only heating effects at the tip, or a combination of minimal laser/and mostly hot tip effect. They may be placed over a guidewire, or used on their own. The laser energy makes the metal tip so hot in the front, that it vaporizes away obstructions with some damage to the sidewalls. It is being used in other applications besides laser angioplasty.

The Nd:YAG sapphire contact probes are used in a similar fashion, using a combination of focused laser and heat energy. Recent work suggests this technique causes less tissue damage, is technically easier and more potent than the metal tip, in vascular recanalization.

Excimer lasers have received much attention for laser angioplasty with few clinical trials. The 193 nm wavelength of the argon fluoride (ArFl) excimer would be ideal because of the absence of thermal injury. However fibers are not yet available for this wavelength. The krypton fluoride (KrFl) laser at 248 nm is a possibility, except it has proven mutagenic effects. The xenon chloride (XeCl) laser at 308 nm passes through conventional fibers and is not mutagenic. This XeCl laser will most likely be the excimer of choice for initial vascular work. The light takes just a small 'bite' with each pulse and exhibits less heating effect on the vessel.

Photodynamic therapy

Photodynamic therapy (PDT) involves the use of a photosensitizing agent to treat malignant tumors. In this instance dihematoporphyrin ether (DHE) is the photosensitizing drug used and is activated by 630 nm (red) light produced from an argon pumped dye laser. A hematoporphyrin derivatve (HpD) was used previously, but DHE has been found to be more effective. Other photosensitizing agents are being investigated which include pheophorbide A activated in the Nd:YAG laser wavelength. The laser is used because of its ability to produce intense levels of monochromatic light. Other light sources may be used, such filtered slide projectors, but these are not as effective. The red light from gold and copper vapor lasers is being examined as an alternative light source.

Fluorescence of some tumors upon illumination with a Wood's lamp was noted as long ago as 1924. This principle was then used as a localization technique by the systemic injection of hematoporphyrin, beginning in 1942. Lipson later reported the use of hematoporphyrin derivative which was shown to have a superior tumor localization to that of hematoporphyrin. The use of HpD then moved from diagnostic to therapeutic applications when Diamond reported in 1972, the destruction of experimental tumors by white light exposed after HpD injection. Dougherty's group at Roswell Park Memorial Institute has been studying the response of a wide variety of malignant tumors in man to PDT with various photosensitizers. He reported complete or partial response of 111 out of 113 cutaneous and subcutaneous malignant lesions in 1978.

From the results obtained by various investigators, it appears that PDT is a valid treatment. The DHE is initially distributed through all the cells but begins to clear out of normal tissue after several hours. An initial dose is injected as a single intravenous bolus. A maximum difference in concentration levels between tumor cells and normal cells occurs in about three days. Normal tissue does however, retain some DHE and this is complicated by the fact that different tissues retain various concentrations. Skin, liver, kidney and spleen hold onto the DHE longer than other tissues. Bronchial mucosa retains one of the lowest concentrations and so endobronchial tumors are among the easiest to treat.

The goal of dosimetry is to calculate dosages of drug and light for which activation of the higher concentrations of DHE occurs in cancer cells while remaining below the necessary threshold to activate lower concentrations of DHE in normal tissue. This is

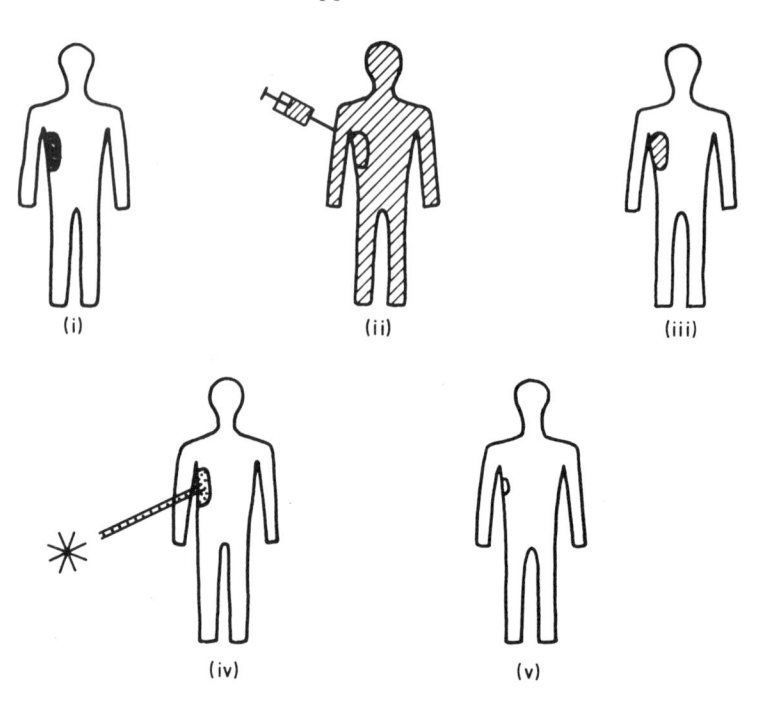

Fig. 20 Diagrammatic and simplified illustration of photoradiation therapy: (i) patient with tumor in chest; (ii) hematoporphyrin derivative (HpD) injected intravenously and taken up by the whole body; (iii) HpD selectively retained by the tumor after about three days; (iv) HpD photoactivated by 630 nm laser light; (v) toxic products produced in (iv) destroy tumor, leaving normal tissues undamaged.

controlled by dosage and timing of the DHE injection, color, intensity and distribution of the light, and its method of delivery. The technique is illustrated diagramatically in Fig. 20, and a patient undergoing treatment is shown in Color Plate I.

Until recently, most patients treated with this form of therapy have previously exhausted the full range of conventional therapies of surgery, radiation, immunotherapy and chemotherapy. Results have been encouraging enough for some investigators to utilize PDT for early lesions as the primary form of treatment.

The absorption spectrum of DHE has peaks which may be utilized to activate the drug. Blue light of about 405 nm is absorbed most strongly but a lesser absorption peak also exists in the range of red light at 630 nm. The red light, however, will penetrate tissue much better than the blue. Red light will scatter up to approximately 2 cm through skin. The amount of light energy delivered to an area is measured with a radiometer and time is calculated to deliver doses of between 25 joules/cm^2 and 150 joules/cm^2, depending on the tumor.

The drug is activated by the light through singlet oxygen production. The vessels of the tumor's blood supply are implicated strongly in the phototoxic process. Gross tissue effects proceed from moderate or severe edema to complete necrosis of the tumor exhibited by a black eschar.

PDT is still investigational and has not been proven as a cure for most malignancies. It will in all probability be used as an adjuvant therapy and, for some neoplasms, the primary form of treatment. Its mechanism is independent of previous or subsequent chemotherapy and/or X-ray therapy.

There are side effects and complications to this form of treatment. Patients undergo an increased photosensitivity of the skin to sunlight for about one month after treatment. Full thickness necrosis of tumors of the intestinal tract may lead to fistula formation. Endobronchial treatments may cause production of gelatinous secretions and edema of the airway causing obstructions. Post treatment hemorrage is possible following necrosis of tumor and any vessels involved.

Current technology with lasers and fiberoptics makes it feasible to deliver high intensity light to almost any site in the body, at surgery, or through endoscopes and needles. Applications include pulmonary, urological, gastrointestinal, ENT and dermatological tumors. PDT may then be used to treat malignancies that are not responsive to current modalities. It may be used to treat nonresectable lesions of the pancreas or brain. Combination therapies with systemic treatment, ionizing radiation or hyperthermia are possible since PDT is a local treatment.

Laserthermia® or interstitial local hyperthermia

The Nd.YAG laser used in combination with contact interstitial endoprobes and temperature sensors has been used to treat cancer both experimentally and clinically. The tumor tissue is heated to between 42 and 44°C for 20–30 minutes using computer controlled equipment. Over several days tumors necrose, leaving normal tissue. Applications include open, endoscopic and percutaneous placement of probes. Combination therapy with PDT appears synergistic.

6 Laser Safety

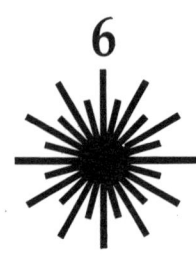

General points

Hazards associated with the use of surgical laser systems require appropriate safety precautions and policies. It is beyond the scope of this section to delineate fully the potential biological and ocular hazards associated with the full spectrum of laser wavelengths. A suggested reading list is included at the end of the book for those who would like more comprehensive information.

The following discusses practical safety considerations as they relate to the surgical or outpatient environment, with carbon dioxide, argon (or KTP) and Nd:YAG laser systems. There is a great deal of overlap in safety practices with these three lasers, with eye protection being the biggest differentiating factor.

Laser manufacturers are required under the ANSI-Z-136.1 standard in the USA and the BSI standard, BS 4803, in the United Kingdom to provide certain design and engineering safety measures in their equipment. In the USA, expressed or implied warranties of merchantibility may not be abrogated by a manufacturer if service is provided on the equipment by third-party service agents. In other countries equivalent conditions may be observed. Safety requirements include provision for such items as key interlocks and visual or audible warning systems. All of the required measures are in place on commercially available lasers and the user need not be concerned with complying with these requirements.

While there is broad international agreement over safety levels and practices involving the use of lasers, differences exist between national administrative mechanisms for accrediting doctors for laser work.

In the United Kingdom, a local body such as the Radiological Safety Committee is concerned with laser safety policy, but does not take upon itself responsibility for accrediting laser users.

However, the British Medical Laser Association (BMLA) has been asked to consider accreditation in individual cases.

In the USA, no medical or governmental agency credentials doctors for laser use. Doctors are credentialed through their medical license and respective specialty boards to practice medicine. Laser is simply a surgical tool used in the practice of medicine. The American Society for Laser Medicine and Surgery (ASLMS) of Wausau, Wisconsin also does not credential physicians, however they do provide recommendations on training, suggested before clinical laser use.

The American Board of Laser Surgery offers board examinations for laser use and provides credentialing certificates. This is a private company and is not associated with the American Medical Association (AMA) and its speciality credentialing boards. The objective of this organization is to provide some type of evaluation process for hospitals as a basis for granting laser privileges to physicians. In the sense that it has identified a deficit area in evaluation of physicians knowledge of laser use, its efforts are worthwhile. Board certification by this company is not required for laser use in the United States. The question of physician evaluation will best be confronted when the true medical specialty boards start including laser-related questions in their board examinations.

Common practice includes the establishment of a Laser Safety Committee with representatives from each of the interested specialties, anesthesiology, operating room director, and administration. This committee can adopt their own credentialing standards for surgeons and establish formal laser safety policies and procedures. Initially this committee is formed to evaluate laser equipment for purchase.

Training is the single most important factor in the safe use of any laser. This applies to surgeons, laser specialists, and operating room personnel.

Customary credentialing standards for physicians include a 12–16 hour hands-on training experience with the laser. This is broken down into three primary areas of experience:

1. Fundamentals of laser surgery (theory)
2. Laboratory hands-on animal work (in most cases)
3. Clinical orientation to procedures in that specialty.

Additionally, some committees require an in-house preceptor for the surgeon's first one or two cases. Once a surgeon is credentialed on a particular type of laser, they should not necessarily have to repeat the entire course for different lasers. Some type of supervized, hands-on orientation to the new type of laser should be sufficient.

Several nurses or surgical technicians may be selected to receive thorough training in the operation and safety practices of the laser. These will be the laser specialists. A laser manufacturer's inservicing of how to operate that particular unit should be complemented with more thorough instruction in the theory of the primary surgical lasers, nursing considerations, and safety practices.

Lasers operated in the simpler environment of an office or clinic may not require dedicated specialists to run the laser. Often the physician or staff in the room can easily do this.

In surgery, laser specialists operate the equipment. The circulator should not be used for this purpose if they must frequently leave the room. The function of the laser specialist is to ensure that hospital personnel follow recommended safety practices, wear the correct protective eyewear, and follow established procedure. The laser should always be placed in the standby position when the surgeon is not using it. If applicable, the laser nurse will also ensure that the physician is on the approved list for laser privileges from the safety committee. The laser specialist will precheck the laser to ensure its proper operation and may maintain a laser log for all cases. This log does not become part of the patient's chart. The physician will chart whatever laser remarks are appropriate, if any, in their operative report.

Operating room personnel need to be instructed in safety procedures relevant to the type of laser used, but need not be taught the detailed operation of the units.

Warning signs should be placed on all entries to the surgical suite before the laser is operated. The signs, which are commercially available, should state the type and class of laser used, and its maximum power.

The keys to the laser should be controlled by the laser specialist, or unit management. The keys should not be left in the lasers. This will control unauthorized access.

Electrical hazards are shared by all types of lasers, as for any electrical equipment. Lasers contain high voltage power supplies and panels should only be removed by trained personnel. Liquids should not be placed on the units because of the potential of spills and resulting short circuiting of the laser. Special cartilages are used for coaxial water applications.

The radiation hazards of the laser, posted on the warning signs, have nothing to do with X-rays or any type of diffuse ionizing radiation around the equipment. The light itself is the radiation referred to. Apart from eye safety, this beam is only a hazard upon direct impact, which would cause a thermal burn. Women in any stage of pregnancy may work around conventional laser units with no adverse effects. An X-ray laser does exist, but is a star wars variety high power laser of interest primarily to the military.

Carbon dioxide lasers

This is currently the most common laser used in an operating room. This wavelength is outside the retinal hazard region because diffuse reflections are not transmitted into the eye. It does present the potential for corneal or scleral burns (or burns anywhere on the body) when the beam is sufficiently focused. The effect is both immediate and painful. For this reason safety glasses are required by all surgical personnel. Either glass or plastic lenses will absorb a diffuse carbon dioxide laser beam. Common practice in a surgery setting is to wear one's own corrective glasses. Side shields are available for additional protection if desired, but are not really necessary. Personnel working in the field, close to the focused beam may simply wish to wear the plastic safety glasses over their own glasses if the additional side protection is desired. Some outpatient clinics have opted to make the glasses available, but optional, for personnel in the room because of the relative safety of using these units, especially when attached to a colposcope. Contact lenses of any type are inadequate. In the United Kingdom, ordinary safety glasses would be considered inadequate, as they do not conform to the requirements of the Protection of Eye Regulations 1974. The lenses in any microscope or rigid endoscope serve as the protection for the operating surgeon.

The patient's eyes must also be protected if they are in a position that exposes them to the laser. Wet sponges taped in place over the eyes if the patient is asleep, or safety glasses if they are awake, will provide protection.

Sponges and drapes are also kept moist for fire protection. These materials are soaked only in the immediate surgical field. Dry sponges will flame immediately upon impact with the carbon dioxide laser. A container of water or saline should always be kept available to douse a flame if needed. The normal pan of irrigation solution will serve this purpose.

Most paper drapes available in the USA are fire resistant and may be safely used with the laser. Cloth drapes may have moist sponges draped at the perimeter of the field. A drape will flame only if it is directly impacted with the laser beam.

Do not use the laser in the presence of flammable preparative solutions or drying agents. This is most important for the carbon dioxide laser but would apply to any type. These preparative solutions may be used on the patient, but the area should be dry before lasing.

During oral, nasopharyngeal or laryngotracheal surgery, special precautions must be taken to avoid an airway explosion and blowtorch type of fire. Though foil tape protection is of primary importance, polyvinylchloride (PVC) endotracheal tube must *never* be used during this type of surgery. Alternatives include Norton flexible metal tubes, red rubber tubes wrapped with foil tape, or laser resistant tubes available from several manufacturers.

When the Norton tubes are used, no distal cuff is used, so that no flammable materials rest in the airway. This provides complete protection against fire but leaves an open ventilation system. If sized well, they provide a good fit and leak very little.

Red rubber tubes are wrapped in an overlapping spiral fashion from the cuff up with reflective foil tape. Each batch of tape should be tested to ensure that the laser will not penetrate. After intubation, the inflated cuff is packed off well with moist cottonoids. The cuff may be inflated with saline and methylene blue dye. If the cuff were inadvertently ruptured, the blue saline would soak through and the surgeon would be aware of the deflation.

Several new tubes are now commercially available and manufacturer's recommendations should be followed in using laser resistant type tubes. It would still be helpful to inflate the cuff with fluid and seal off the end with moist packing.

Jet ventilation for microlaryngeal laser surgery is an excellent alternative and eliminates flammable material from the airway. None of the tubes should be tightly taped in place during these procedures so that they may be pulled quickly if a fire starts. The tube may be marked with a distance marker to maintain the correct distance. The laser must obviously never be used in the presence of explosive anesthetics.

Methane gas is also flammable. When lasing up into the rectum, it should be packed or covered with a moist towel or sponge. Failure to do so could cause serious internal injury to the patient and/or facial burns to the surgeon.

During microlaryngoscopies, or when otherwise exposing the patient's face to the laser beam, the entire face should be draped with wet towels. The only exposed area should be the oral cavity. Care should be taken to protect the teeth with bite blocks or soaked sponges. A carbon dioxide laser impact on tooth enamel will create a small, permanent, black hole in the tooth.

Special instrumentation is available that has been blackened or anodized to reduce the danger of the beam reflecting off the instrument and striking other objects. These instruments are an important safety precaution for microlaryngoscopy. They are of benefit, but not critical, in other types of carbon dioxide laser surgery. It is the diffuse matt finish of the instrument rather than the black color that reduces reflection. When regular retractors are being used, they may be covered with moistened sponges for protection. Teflon coated instruments should not be used in a laser field as they produce toxic fumes when lased.

Pyrex, quartz, or titanium rods are routinely used in gynecologic laser surgery as fine dissecting rods and backstops. Glass rods should not be used because they will shatter, leaving tiny glass fragments in the field.

Nd:YAG lasers

Safety precautions center around eye safety and care of endoscopes. Fire precautions must still be taken, but this is not as much of a hazard here as with the carbon dioxide laser.

It is critically important that all personnel are wearing the appropriate safety glasses *before* they enter the room when the laser is being fired. Regular glasses will not suffice. Until recently Nd:YAG safety glasses were green or green-gray colored, new clear glasses for clarity of vision are now available. All safety glasses are marked as to the wavelength covered, as well as the optical density of the material. It is very important to look at the wavelength markings on these safety glasses before putting them on. If one did not look at the markings for 1060 nm (or 1.06 micron) to cover the Nd:YAG, it would be possible to get the glasses mixed up. Safety goggles, glasses or clip-on lenses are designed to fit over one's own corrective glasses. Prescription laser safety glasses are available for purchase. Eyepiece filters are available to fit over the end of endoscopes so that the endoscopist need not wear safety glasses. It is important that anyone viewing through a teaching head also have eye protection. It is a common safety practice for all personnel in the room to wear protective eyewear during endoscopy, even though they are not actually at risk when the laser is fired only in this closed environment. Video-endoscopy removes the need for eye-protection for both medical staff and patient. With the use of contact probes, the combination of the probe and low powers significantly reduces potential eye hazards, however protective eyewear is still recommended but at much lower optical densities.

As with any laser, it is possible to install door interlocks that will automatically shut off the laser when the door is opened. The use of these door interlocks in a surgery setting should be discouraged. Instead the fact that training is the single most important factor in the safe use of any laser should be reasserted.

Windows in the room should be covered in open surgery so that observers are protected from unintentional viewing. Panels may be made for the windows, or towels may simply be taped over them. Patients' eyes are protected by covering with towels or sponges. Patients who are awake should wear protective eyewear.

Operating microscopes do not provide eye protection for the Nd:YAG laser and the surgeon must either wear protective eyewear, or a filter incorporated into the manipulator device. Room personnel must all wear protective eyewear.

It is possible to cause extensive damage, or total destruction, to flexible endoscopes by firing the laser with the fiber not fully extended from the channel. This is possible because one can still see the guide light on the target while the fiber is still within the scope. As a matter of policy, it is important for the surgeon to have the tip of the fiber in his field of view before firing the laser. A distance of 1.0–2.0 cm is an adequate distance from the scope.

Because of the high degree of back scatter with the non-contact Nd:YAG laser, and the dark color of the tip of most endoscopes, it is possible to melt this tip and even cause a small fire if high concentrations of oxygen are used, as in bronchoscopy. The further away from the tip the fiber is placed, the better.

A fire hazard also exists when lasing an airway tumor while ventilating with high concentrations of oxygen, this is reduced with contact YAG laser surgery and coaxial water. Fat in a tumor may flare from the laser and, in the presence of oxygen, cause a small flash. Though undesirable, this does not pose the risk and types of problems associated with an endotracheal tube fire from the carbon dioxide laser. Entrainment of air into the ventilating gas is sometimes used to maintain lower (less than 40%) oxygen concentrations. The use of pulse oxymeters allows the lowest, safest oxygen concentrations.

In ophthalmic applications the beams of the Nd:YAG laser (photodisruptors) are generally focused at a large angle of convergence, so that beyond the focus the beam intensity drops quickly. However, reflections from the surface of the cornea or the contact lens can still be hazardous up to a meter or so away, depending on the curvature of the reflecting surface. Therefore, it is important that attendant staff wear safety glasses when treatments are in progress.

Argon and KTP lasers

Essentially, the wavelengths on these lasers are close enough that safety glasses and precautions are identical. The exception is a special safety glass which the KTP manufacturer has designed to such a narrow bandwidth to be useful for only this laser. The discussion of argon also implies application to KTP.

The argon lasers are used through either a handpiece, microscope, bare fiber, or slit lamp. In some ophthalmic equipment they are used in conjunction with a krypton laser. KTP is rarely used through slit lamps.

These lasers present almost no fire hazard, and eye protection is the central safety requirement. Special orangish colored glasses for the argon wavelength must be worn by all personnel in the room. Argon and KTP present potential retinal hazards. As with Nd:YAG, covers should be placed over the room windows and the patient's eyes should be covered or they should wear the glasses. It is important to check the label on the glasses to determine the wavelength covered (488 and 515 for the argon and 532 for the KTP) so as not to confuse them with the newer type of Nd:YAG glasses.

The sole manufacturers of the KTP laser for medical use has developed clear safety glasses for use with their laser, which is very convenient. This filter material was designed to cover only the KTP wavelength and not the argon — according to the manufacturers. Clear filter material is possible for argon lasers but as yet is not commercially available for medical use. Depending on the manufacturer, laser attachments for microscopes, slit lamps, and endoscopes have automatic shutter filters that protect the surgeon from the flash of light.

In endoscopic procedures that do not have the automatic shutter filters, it is important to place a filter over the eyepiece or wear safety glasses.

In ophthalmic procedures through the slit lamp, it is still advisable for personnel to wear protective eyewear since specular reflections at certain angles from the slit lamp may be picked up by the eye.

All laser procedures are safe for both patient and personnel provided one acquires proper training, observes necessary precautions, and maintains equipment in proper operating order. Commonsense is the most important factor in safety.

Further Reading

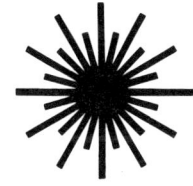

Absten, G.T. (1988) *The Myth of Lasers in Medicine*, Advanced Laser Services Corporation, Columbus, OH.

Joffe, S.N. (1988) *Lasers in General Surgery*, Williams and Wilkins, Baltimore, MD.

Lanzafame, R. and Hinshaw, J.R. (1988) *Atlas of CO_2 Laser Surgical Techniques*, Ishiyaku EuroAmerica, St Louis, MO.

Sanfilippo, J.S. and Levine, R.L. (1988) *Gynecologic Endoscopy, Pelviscopic Surgery and Laser Laparoscopy*, Springer-Verlag, NY.

Laser Focus/Penwell Publications, *1988 Medical Laser Buyers Guide*, Littleton, MA.

Minton, J.P. and Absten, G.T. (Feb. 1987) *Surgical Lasers – and How they Work*, American College of Surgeons Bulletin.

Absten, G.T. (1987) *Evaluation of Surgical Laser Technology*, Advanced Laser Services Corp., Columbus, OH.

Absten, G.T. (1987) *Laser Techniques of Tomorrow*, Middle East Health Magazine, London, England.

Apfelberg, D. (1987) *Evaluation and Installation of Surgical Laser Systems*, Springer-Verlag, NY.

Fuller, T.A. (1987) *Surgical Lasers, A Clinical Guide*, Macmillan Publishing Co., NY.

Absten, G.T. (1986) *Fundamentals of Laser Surgery*, Advanced Laser Services Corp., Columbus, OH.

Martin, D.C., Absten, G.T., Levinson, C.J. and Photopulos, G.J. (1986) *Intra-Abdominal Laser Surgery*, Resurge Press, Memphis, TN.

Ratz, J.L. (1986) *Lasers in Cutaneous Medicine and Surgery*, Year Book Medical Publishers, Chicago, IL.

American National Standard for the Safe Use of Lasers, ANSI 2136.1 (1986) American National Standards Institute, NY.

Belcher, C.D., Thomas, J.V. and Simmons, R.J. (1984) *Photocoagulation in Glaucoma and Anterior Segment Disease*, Waverly Press Inc, Baltimore, MD.

Further Reading

Mackety, C. (1984) *Perioperative Laser Nursing*, Slack Inc, Thorofare, NJ.

March, W. (1984) *Ophthalmic Lasers: Current Clinical Uses*, Slack Inc, Thorofare, NJ.

Andrews, A. and Polyani, T. (1982) *Microscopic and Endoscopic Surgery with the CO_2 Laser*, Wright PSG Inc, Boston, MA.

Maurer, A. (1982) *Lasers: Light Wave of the Future*, Arco Publishing, NY.

Goldman, L. (1981) *The Biomedical Laser: Technology and Clinical Applications*, Springer-Verlag, NY.

Johnson, J. (1981) *A Look Inside Lasers*, Raintree Publishers, Milwaukee, WI.

Calder, N. (1979) *Einstein's Universe*, Viking Press, NY.

Hallmark, C. (1979) *Lasers, The Light Fantastic*, Tab Books, Blue Ridge Summit, PA.

Goldman, L. (1967) *Biomedical Aspects of the Laser*, Springer-Verlag, NY.

Einsten, A. (1961) *Relativity*, Bonanza Books, NY.

Einstein, A. (1954) *Ideas and Opinions*, Bonanza Books, NY.

Laser Institute of America (1983) *Laser Safety Guide*, Toledo, OH.

U.S. Dept of Health, Education and Welfare Public Health Service, Food and Drug Administration, *Biological Bases for and Other Aspects of a Performance Standard for Laser Products*, HEW Publication (FDA) 80–8092.

Index

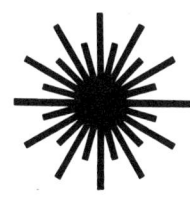

Abdominal cysts 35
Absorption 17, 18, 19
Acne 41
Acoustic neuromas 40
Adenomas, recurrent 40
Adhesions 35, 36
Advantages, laser surgery 34
Aiming beam, laser 33
Airfiber, *see* Waveguide delivery systems
Airway, explosion risk 58
Airway lesions 38, 39
Airway tumors, fire hazards with 60
Alexandrite laser 10
Ali method, hemorrhoids 43
Amalgam, laser preparation for 45
Amenorhea 37
American National Standards Institute (ANSI), standard for laser manufacturer 54
Amplitude 2
Anastomosis 49–50
Anesthetics, explosion risk from 60
Angioma, Campbell DeMorgan senile 41
Angiomata, gastrointestinal 43
Angioplasty 26, 50
Animal work, training by 55
Argon laser 9, 13, 16, 17, 23, 24
  delivery systems 29–30, 33
  dermatologic and plastic surgery applications 41, 42
  gastroenterology applications 42
  gynecologic applications 35, 37
  ophthalmic applications 46–8
  otorhinolaryngology applications (ENT) 37, 38
  safety of 61
  special safety glasses for 59, 61
  urological applications 44
  vascular applications 43, 49, 50
Argon pumped dye lasers 50
Argon fluoride laser 9, 10, 21, 26, 30, 49, 50
Arteriotomies, welding of 49
Arteriovenous malformations (AVM's) 39
Arthroscopy 46
Articulated arms 7, 27, 30, 35
Artificial joints 46
Asherman's syndrome 37
Atomic processes 4

Back scatter 18, 60
Back surgery 40–1
Bladder surgery 44
Blood flow, as heat sink 20
Bone cutting 21
Brain surgery 39–41
Breast surgery 42
British Medical Laser Association (BMLA) 55
British Standards Institution (BSI), standard for laser manufacturer 54
Bronchoscopes 29, 38, 39, 60
Burns
  debridement of 45
  facial 58

66 Index

Capillary/cavernous hemangiomas 41
Carbon dioxide (CO$_2$) lasers 9, 10, 16, 18, 20–3, 34
   delivery systems 27–9
   dermatologic and plastic surgery applications 41, 42
   flowing gas systems 11
   general surgery applications 45
   gynecologic applications 35, 36
   neurosurgical applications 39, 40
   ophthalmic applications 46
   oral surgery and dental applications 45
   orthopedic applications 46
   otorhinolaryngology (ENT) applications 37, 38
   safety of 57–9
   sealed tube systems 10, 11
   urological applications 43, 44
   vascular applications 49
Carbon monoxide laser 10
Caries, dental 45
Cartilage, cutting 20–1
Cataract surgery 48
Cavities, *see* Caries
Cervical Intraepithelial Neoplasia (CIN) 36
Cervical surgery 36
Char 18, 20, 22, 23, 42
Choanal atresia 38
Clinical applications 34
   dermatology and plastic surgery 41, 42
   gastroenterology 42, 43
   general surgery 45
   gynecology 35–7
   neurosurgery 39–41
   oral surgery and dentistry 45
   orthopedics 46
   ophthalmology 46–9
   photodynamic therapy 50–3
   pulmonary 38, 39
   urology 43, 44
   vascular 49, 50
Coagulation 16, 18, 20, 25

Coaxial gas delivery 29, 30, 32, 43
Coaxial fluid delivery 32, 43
Coherence 3, 4, 6–8
Collagen production, reduction by Nd:YAG laser 42
Collimation 8
Colposcopic procedures 36
Computer laser scanners 29
Condyloma 36
Cone angle 48
Contact lenses 57
Contact probes
   diamond 25
   quartz 25
   see also Sapphire probes
Corneal burns, danger of 57
Corneal incisions 26, 49
Corneal sculpting 49
Corneal transplants 49
Cornual implants 36
Copper vapor laser 9
Coupling cube, laser 35, 38
Cranial tumors 40
Craniotomy 40
Credentialling of surgeons 54–6
Cryosurgery, heavy discharge from 36
Cryosurgery, hemorrhoid treatment 43
Cutting 16, 18, 20–2, 25, 26
Cystoscopes 44

Debridement
   burns 45
   decubitus ulcers 45
Defocused beams 22, 23, 28, 29
Delivery systems 27–33
Dental applications 26, 45
Dermatology 41, 42
Diabetic retinopathy 47
Dihematoporphyrin ether (DHE) 50–2
Dilantin hyperplasia 45
Diskectomy 40, 41
Disruptive effects 15, 48
Dorsal root entry zone (DREZ) lesions 40

Index

Dougherty PhD, Thomas 51
Dye lasers 9, 10, 25
  argon pumped 50, 51
  delivery systems 30
  dermatology applications 25, 26, 41
  ophthalmic applications 25
  photodynamic therapy applications 50, 51
Dysphagia, palliation of 43

Einstein's theories – back cover, 2
Electrical hazards 56
Electrically energized lasers 10
Electromagnetic spectrum 1
Electrons 4–6
Electrosurgical coagulation 20
Endobronchial lung tumors 39, 51
Endometrial ablation 37
Endometriosis 35
Endoscopes 29, 33, 38, 39, 42–4, 53, 60
Endotracheal tubes 58
Energy 12
Energy density, *see* Fluence
Erbium Yttrium Aluminum Garnet (Er:YAG) lasers 21
Esophageal varices 43
Excimer lasers 9, 26, 21, 49
Explosion risks 58
Extracorporeal shock wave lithotripsy (EWSL) 44
Eye protection 57, 59–61
Eye surgery 46–9

Fallopian tube procedures 35, 36
Fenestration, syringomyelia 40
Fiber, CO_2 laser 27
  see also Waveguide delivery system
Fiberoptic systems 27–33
Filling, *see* Amalgam
Filters, endoscopes 59, 61
Fire hazards 21, 57–60
Fire protection 21, 57–60
First medical laser uses 46

Fistula formation 43, 53
Flammable agents 58
Flash fires 60
Flexible endoscopes 39, 42, 50, 53, 60
Fluence 12
Fluorescence 51
Focal length 7, 12, 22–3, 28, 29, 39
Focused beams 8, 12, 13, 20, 22–3, 28–9
Food and Drug Administration (FDA–USA) 41, 45
Frequency 2
Frequency doubled Nd:YAG laser 24
  see also KTP laser
Fundamentals of laser surgery 1–33, 55

Gas lasers 10
Gastroenterology 42, 43
Gastrointestinal bleeding 42, 43
General surgery 45
Genital lesions 36, 44
Gingivectomy 45
Glass rods 59
Glaucoma treatment 47, 48
Gold vapor lasers 9, 51
Granuloma 37
Gum tissue, sculpting 45
Gynecology 35–7

Handpieces 28, 29
Hazards 54, 56–61
  long focal length 39
Heater probes 42, 43
Heating, absorptive 16
Helium neon (HeNe) lasers 9, 10, 33
Hematoporphyrin derivative (HpD) 50, 51
Hemoglobin, absorption by 24, 26
Hemophilia patients 38
Hemorrhoids 43
Hemostatic effects 16, 18, 20, 25, 34
Hertz (Hz) units 2
Hollow waveguide, *see* Waveguide delivery system
Hot tips 50

Hydrogen fluoride (HF) laser 10
Hyperthermia, combined therapy 53
Hypertrophic scarring 42
Hypophysectomy 40
Hysterectomies, alternative to 37
Hysteroscope procedures 37

Incoherence 3–5, 7, 8
Independent laser service 54
Infraguide, *see* Waveguide
Infrared lasers 9, 21
 see also Carbon dioxide; Nd:YAG; Er:YAG
Interlocks, door/key 54, 60
Intractable pain 40
Intramedullary tumors 40
Intraocular lens (IOL) 48
Ionization effect 48
Ionizing radiation, combined treatment 53
Iridectomy 48
Iridotomy 47, 48
Irradiance 12

Jet ventilation 58
Joules 12

Keloid scars 42
Keys, laser 54, 56
Kidney procedures 44
Kidney stones 44
Krypton lasers 9, 10
 ophthalmic applications 47
Krypton fluoride lasers 9, 26, 50
KTP lasers 9, 16, 24, 25, 29, 30, 33, 35, 37, 38, 41, 43, 61, 62
 see also Argon lasers

Laboratory training 55
Laparoscopes 29, 35
Laryngeal diseases 37, 38
Laser, acronym 1
 light
  properties of 7–9
  tissue effects of 16–21
 logbook 56

medium 9, 10
physics 1–15
plume 18, 19
resistant endotracheal tubes 58
safety 54–62
safety committee 55
tubes, refurbishment of 46
Leukoplakia 38
Liability, manufacturer's 54
Light, nature of 1
Lipson M.D. 51
Liquid lasers 9, 10
Lithotripsy
 extracorporeal shock wave (eswl) 44
 laser 26, 30, 44
Liver metastases 45
Lymphostatic effects 42, 44

Macula 46, 47
Maintenance, of lasers 54, 62
Malignancies 50–3
Manufacturer's product liability 54
Manufacturers, safety requirements for 54
Mastectomy 42
Matt finish, instrumentation 59
Melanin, absorption by 24
Mengiomas, vaporizing of 40
Menorrhagia 29
Metal endotracheal tubes 58
Methane gas, flammability 58
Methyl methacrylate glue 38
 see also Polymethyl methacrylate (PMM)
Microlaryngoscopy 37–8, 58, 59
Micromanipulator 28, 29, 33
Microscopes, operating 28
Microsurgery, orthopedic 46
Microtuboplasty 35–6
Mirror, partially reflective 7
Mirrors, articulated arm 27
Mode locked lasers 15
 ophthalmic applications 48, 49
Modes 13–15
Molecular processes 10, 11

Moles 41
Monochromatic light sources 51
Monochromaticity 9
Mutagenic effects 26, 50
Myringotomy 38

Nanometer 2
Neodymium gadolinium aluminum scandium garnet (Nd:GASG) laser 10
Neodymium glass (Nd:glass) laser 9
Neodymium yttrium aluminum garnet (Nd:YAG) lasers 9, 18, 20, 25
  delivery systems 30–3
  dermatology applications 41
  gastroenterology applications 42–3
  general surgery applications 45
  neurosurgical applications 39, 40
  ophthalmic applications 46–9
  oral surgery and dental applications 45
  orthopedic applications 46
  otorhinolaryngology (ENT) applications 38
  pulmonary applications 38, 39
  safety of 59–61
  urologic applications 43, 44
  vascular applications 49–50
Neosalpingotomy 36
Nephrectomy, partial 44
Nerves, rejoining of 46
Neurosurgery 39–41
Nevi 41
Norton metal endotracheal tubes 58
Nurses, training of 56

Office procedures 36, 44, 47
Operating microscopes, safety of 57, 60
Operating room personnel 55–7, 59–62
Ophthalmic applications 15, 25, 30, 46–9, 60–1
Ophthalmology 23, 25, 26, 46–9

Optic chiasm, preservation of 40
Optical concepts 12–15
Optical density 59
Oral cavity lesions 38
Orthopedics 21, 26, 46
Otorhinolaryngology 37, 38, 58, 59
Outpatient procedures 36, 47
Overdistension, by cooling gas 43
Oxygen levels, retina 47
Oxygen, hazards with laser 60

Pain, reduced postoperatively 34, 37, 45
Pan-retinal photocoagulation (PRP) 47
Pancreatectomy, partial 45
Paper drapes 57, 58
Papillomas 37, 38
Pediatric surgery 37
Pelvic inflammatory disease (PID) 35
Penile carcinoma 44
Peptic ulcers 42
Perforation 39
Phase 3, 6–8
Photodisruption 48
  see also Sonic effects; Ionization effects; Disruptive effects
Photodynamic therapy (PDT) 26, 50–3
Photolysis 26
Photons 1, 4–6
Photosensitivity 50, 51, 53
Phototoxic effect 52
Physics, laser 1–15
Pigment epithelium 47
Pigmented tissue 24
Plastic surgery 41, 42
Policies, laser 54, 55
Polyps 37
Polymethylmethacrylate (PMM) glue 46
  see also Methylmethacrylate
Polyvinylchloride (PVC) endotracheal tubes 58
Population inversion 4, 6

Portwine hemangiomas 24, 41
Portwine stains 24, 41
Posterior capsulotomy 48
Power 28, 30, 33, 40, 43, 49, 56, 60
    factors affecting 2, 3, 7, 8, 11, 12, 27
    units of 12
    values quoted 11, 12, 15, 18, 24, 25, 30, 36, 39, 45, 48, 49
Power density 12, 18, 27–9, 31, 36, 44, 46
    measurement of 12
    values quoted 12, 49, 52
    see also Energy density
Preceptorship 55
Pregnancy, laser not a hazard 57
Procedures, laser 55, 56
Properties, individual lasers 22–6
Prostate cancer 44
Prostatectomy 44
Protection of Eye Regulation 1974 (UK) 57
Protective eyewear 56, 57, 59–61
Pulsed lasers 15, 24, 25, 26, 41, 44, 47–50
Pulsing 23, 26, 38, 39, 40, 41, 45, 49
Pumping, result of 4
Pyogenic granuloma 41
Pyrex rods 59

Q-switched lasers 24, 30–5, 46
    ophthalmic applications 47–9
Q-switching 15
Quartz rods 59

Radiation hazards 57
Radical vulvectomies 36
Radio frequency (RF) waveguide CO_2 lasers 10, 11
Radiological Safety Committee 54
Rectum lasing, fire risk 58
Reflecting surfaces 59
Reflection 17
Respiratory papillomatosis 37, 38
Red rubber endotracheal tubes 58
Retina, photocoagulation of 23, 47

Retractors 59
Rhinophyma 38
Ruby lasers 9

Safety factors 54–62
Sapphire (contact) probes 22, 25, 30–3, 36, 38, 39, 42–6, 50
Scattering 16–18, 52, 60
Scleral burns, danger of 57
Scleral flaps 46
Scleral tumors 46
Sealed tube, argon laser 24
Sealed tube CO_2 lasers 10, 11
Sebaceous nevi 41
Senile macular degeneration (SMD) 47
Service agents 54
Side shields, on eyewear 57
Singlet oxygen production 52
Skin flaps 42
Slit lamps 29, 46, 47
Solid state lasers 9, 10
Sonic effects 15, 26, 48
    see also Ionization effects
Specular reflections 59, 61
Spinal tumors 40
Sponges
    flammability of 57
    wetted for eye protection 57
Spontaneous emission 4, 5
Spot sizes 8, 12–14, 18, 23, 28, 38, 48, 49
Standby position 56
Stapedotomy 38
Star Wars laser 57
Sterile field production 34, 42, 45
Stimulated emission 4, 6, 7
Strawberry marks 41
Sunlight, sensitivity to 53
Sunlight, laser brighter than 8
Superpulse 20–2, 38
Surgical technicians, training of 56
Sutures, cutting of internal 48
Synechia 38
Syringomyelia 40

Tattoos 41, 42
Teaching head protection, endoscopes 59
Teflon coated instruments 59
Telangiectasias 38, 41
Third party service 54
Tissue fusion, see Welding
Tissue interaction 16–21
Titanium rods 59
Tongue release 38
Tonsillectomy 38
Tooth enamel 45
Tooth enamel, possible damage to 59
Trabeculoplasty 48
Training 55, 56, 60
Transmission 16, 17, 24, 25, 41
Transverse Electromagnetic Mode (TEM) 13–15
Tumors
    abdominal 35
    bladder 43, 44
    cranial 39, 40
    eye 46
    gastrointestinal 43
    intramedullary 40
    lung 38, 39, 51
    photodynamic therapy for 50–3
    spinal 40
    vascular 39, 40
Tunable dye laser, see Dye laser
Turbinectomy 38
Tympanoplasty 38

UK, safety practices 54, 55, 57
Ulcers 42, 43
    debridement of decubitus 45
Ultraviolet lasers 9, 26, 30, 49, 50
Urethral strictures 44
Urology 43, 44

USA, safety practices 54–62
Uterine myomas 36
Uterine septae 36, 37

Vaginal Intraepithelial Neoplasia (VIN) 36
Vaporization 16, 18, 20, 22–5, 31, 45, 50
Varicose veins 41
Vas deferens 44
Vascular surgery 49, 50
Vascular tumors 39, 40
Velocity of light 2
Visual hazards 57, 59–61
Vitreal strands, cutting of 47, 48
Vocal cord applications 37
Vulvectomy 36

Warning signs 54, 56
Warranties, manufacturer's 54
Watts 12
Wave properties 1–3
Waveguide delivery systems, CO_2 laser 27, 28
    see also Fiber, CO_2 laser
Wavelength 1, 2, 13
    characteristic absorption 18, 22, 24, 25, 26, 41, 46, 47, 50, 52
    characteristic of various lasers 9, 22, 24–6
Welding (tissue fusion) 16, 44, 47, 49, 50
Windows, covering of 60
Woods lamp, illumination by 51
Wound healing 22

X-ray lasers 57
Xanthophyll pigment 47
Xenon chloride laser 9, 10, 26, 50